Assessment OF Parenting Competency in Mothers with Mental Illness

Assessment OF Parenting Competency in Mothers with Mental Illness

by

Teresa Ostler, Ph.D.

School of Social Work
University of Illinois at Urbana-Champaign

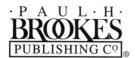
·P·A·U·L·H·
BROOKES
PUBLISHING CO ®

Baltimore • London • Sydney

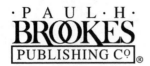

Paul H. Brookes Publishing Co.
Post Office Box 10624
Baltimore, Maryland 21285-0624

www.brookespublishing.com

Typeset by Maryland Composition, Inc., Laurel, Maryland.
Manufactured in the United States of America by
Versa Press, Inc., East Peoria, Illinois.

The case studies in this book are composites based on the authors' experiences.
Names and identifying details have been changed to protect confidentiality.

Library of Congress Cataloging-in-Publication Data

Ostler, Teresa.
  Assessment of parenting competency in mothers with mental illness / by Teresa
Ostler.
    p.   cm.
  ISBN-13: 978-1-55766-665-9
  ISBN-10: 1-55766-665-2
  1. Children of the mentally ill.   2. Mothers—Mental health.   3. Parenting—
Evaluation.   4. Parental influences.   5. Mother and child.   6. Child welfare.
I. Title.
  RJ507.M44O88 2008
  618.92'89—dc22   2007027218

British Library Cataloguing in Publication data are available from the British Library.

Contents

About the Author

Teresa Ostler, Ph.D., Associate Professor, School of Social Work, University of Illinois at Urbana-Champaign, 1207 West Oregon Street, Urbana, IL 61801

Dr. Ostler is a licensed clinical psychologist and received her bachelor of arts degree and doctoral degree in psychology from the University of California at Berkeley in 1973 and 1984, respectively. She joined the School of Social Work at the University of Illinois at Urbana-Champaign as an associate professor in 2003. Prior to this, she was a faculty member in the Department of Psychiatry at the University of Illinois at Chicago and the lead psychologist on the Parenting Assessment Team, a multidisciplinary team that assessed the parenting capabilities of individuals with mental illness who had lost custody of their children. Dr. Ostler's research focuses on parent–child attachment relationships, individuals with major mental illness as parents, children of parents with major mental illness and substance use problems, and children in foster care.

Contributors

Niki Grajewski, M.S.W., QMHP
Southern Illinois Regional Social Services
604 East College
Carbondale, IL 62901

Heather Hasslinger, B.A., M.S.
Jane Addams College of Social Work
University of Illinois at Chicago
9322 3rd Avenue
#195
Brooklyn, NY 11209

Foreword

One of the most challenging clinical tasks is to help decide if a parent–child relationship should be limited or perhaps curtailed. Solomon-like judgment can be required, parceling and balancing competing interests and sometimes inconsistent information to integrate a complex mosaic of conditions and requirements into decisive advice that is meant to divine the future. One is asked to navigate between intruding unnecessarily into a crucial and almost-sacred parent–child relationship but to not leave a child in harm's way with an incapable parent. Missing the mark in either way can cause serious harm to the child as well as the parent. One must determine the best way to support and nurture a crucial relationship while ensuring protection.

Among the most common reasons for such a request of professional service and opinion is the presence of serious mental illness in the mother that is associated with evidence or fear of possible neglect or direct harm to the child. For much of the history of mental health evaluation, clinical practice and related policies have been cast from grant theories of psychopathology and suppositions about the mother–child relationship. The quality of the evaluations rested more on the experience, particular acumen, and careful reasoning of a given clinician than on scientific understanding or a codified approach to assessment and formulation. Inconsistency in basis for decisions as well in what was emphasized in programs and policies was the norm.

For the most part, the presence of mental illness was considered equitable to parental incompetence and potential for child harm. The presumption often was of diminished parenting capacity when mental illness was evident in the primary caregiver. This led to dismissal of the assertion by mothers with mental illness of their ability and commitment to care for their child. At the same time, parents with risky or harmful behavior but deemed to not have mental illness were presumed to have adequate parental skills and often left to care for children despite histories of abuse and neglect. The result was injustice for many: for mothers, for children, and for those wanting to help and care for both.

The pioneering work summarized in *Assessment of Parenting Competency in Mothers with Mental Illness* is instrumental in leading to clear differentiation of mental illness in mothers and child risk for abuse and neglect. The volume is exemplary in helping specify the approach necessary to assess both of these concerns when they overlap. As treatment advances have led to more individuals with mental illness functioning well in many areas of their lives and as research has shown the limited relation between mental illness and danger of harm to others, a need is growing to advance beyond identifying mental illness in the caregiver to understand the functioning of that person and what makes a difference in functional level. Specific to the topic of this book is the need to determine what the parenting situation is and how mental illness in a primary caregiver might be considered thoughtfully and effectively for the well-being of the child.

Dr. Ostler provides here the first sound, empirically based, theoretically integrated, and clinically practical guide for those undertaking such work. By basing the approach, activities, and organization of the assessment in extant research on normal development, parent–child relationships, mental illness effects on caregiving, and which support, treatments, and situations can make a difference in capacity, she gives the interested professional a reliable and useful perspective on what is at stake and what should be considered in undertaking this clinical task. She helps guide the reader through the relative importance and limitations of the science in rendering evaluation of capacity to care adequately and to also consider the costs in constraining or removing the primary caregiver. This volume grounds complex and subtle clinical considerations in the best scientific understanding to replace a prior reverence for some aspect of the multiple influences on development and on effects of major mental illness. Dr. Ostler demonstrates how to translate and organize that scientific understanding into an impressively sensitive and astute feel for the lives being affected by the assessments being requested. She realizes that clinical care derives from our best science, and its most reliable application is the best way to be effective.

This volume will not take the place of sound and extensive training in clinical assessment and mental health. Neither will it provide set answers for the myriad situations that one encounters in trying to determine how best to help a family with a mother with mental illness and a child at risk. It will not compensate for careful listening and attention to the details of a given case. It can, though, guide those undertaking these important and tough clinical responsibilities to provide more reliable and valid assessment and to render with more confidence professional judgment, clinical formulations, and case planning. In doing so, this volume can lead to more justice for those children and families to be assessed in the future.

Patrick Tolan, Ph.D.
Director, Institute for Juvenile Research
Chicago, Illinois

Acknowledgments

This book represents a compilation of my experience in providing parenting assessments and treatment to mothers and fathers with mental illness and in supporting them as they worked to improve their parenting or as they struggled to deal with the grief and pain that accompanies custody loss. These families taught me firsthand about what it means to parent and raise children while having a mental illness.

I also learned much from members of the Parenting Assessment Team at the University of Illinois at Chicago and from the interns and fellows who spent time in working with the team. The Parenting Assessment Team was created in the wake of a highly publicized case in Illinois. In 1993, a mother who had been diagnosed with schizophrenia hanged her young son shortly after he was returned to her care. A special multidisciplinary Mental Health Task Force Special Wallace Case Investigation Team appointed by then Governor Jim Edgar investigated the incident. The task force underscored a lack of communication and methodological soundness in the assessment of parents with mental illness and recommended the creation of an independent assessment team to aid the state child protective services and juvenile court in decision making.

I was fortunate to be part of the independent multidisciplinary team that resulted from the recommendations of this task force. I participated for many years on this team as the lead developmental and clinical psychologist and learned much from the following individuals: Laura Miller, Jesse Reyes, Shane Long, Heather Hasslinger, Joseph Scally, Amy Leventhal, Elena Quintana, Vivien Jones, Marilu Garcia, Grant White, Rosemary Harris, Ralph Moore, Alyssa Slay, Alexandra Ramos, Alissa Levy-Chung, Jackie Haimes, Julia Kim-Cohen, Mrinal Mullick, Chinimayee Barve, and Ane Marinez-Lora.

The following colleagues helped me at various phases of learning and writing: Denise Kane, Mary Ellen Barone, Boris Astrachan, Patrick Tolan, Joseph Flaherty, Marcus Kruesi, John Coverdale, Carl Bell, Judy Stoewe, Geraldine Fox, Karen Budd, Mary Brunette, Wynne S. Korr, Wendy Haight, Barry Ackerson, Megan Kirshbaum, and Joanne Nicholson. My thanks also goes to ZERO TO THREE: National Center for Infants, Toddlers and Families for providing me with a fellowship to support this project and to Jessica Allan, Sarah Shepke, Kathryn M. Sheridan, Sarah L. Couch, and Amy Kopperude for their help in preparing the manuscript for publication.

Throughout its conception and writing, the project benefited greatly from support from my mother, Marian Ostler; my husband, Sid Duke; and my daughter, Johanna Jacobsen Kiciman.

To my father and mother, Bruce and Marian Ostler,
and to my granddaughter, Ella Sibel Kiciman

1

Assessing Parenting in Mothers with Mental Illness

A Daunting Task

Maria became psychotic soon after her first baby was born. Until then, her family had not noted anything unusual about her behavior. In the past weeks, however, troubling changes had occurred in Maria's behavior. In contrast to before, Maria stayed alone in her room for long periods. She refused to talk with others. At times, family members noted her gesturing to the air and conversing with an invisible person. Her family became most alarmed when Maria insisted that she had never given birth to the baby.

Mental health professionals on the psychiatric unit where Maria is hospitalized face hard questions: How long will she remain psychotic? Will psychotropic medication make a difference and, if so, for how long? The most important questions involve potential risks to her baby. What effects will Maria's illness have on the baby's well-being and their developing relationship? Will Maria be able to sustain the stresses of parenting in the days, weeks, and months ahead?

Although many women with mental illness are able to raise their children to adulthood, others may face considerable challenges in the parenting role as they deal with a serious mental illness and the stresses associated with caring for and raising children (Ackerson, 2003; Appleby & Dickens, 1993; Nicholson, Sweeney, & Geller, 1998a). In circumstances in which parenting is compromised, an assessment may be needed to address questions about the impact of a mother's symptoms on her children's well-being and her ability to safely care for them. It will also be necessary to inform interventionists who can help support an individual with mental illness in the parenting role.

Because children of parents with mental illness are at a high risk for both emotional disorders and developmental delays (Beardslee, Versage, & Gladstone, 1998; Brunette & Jacobsen, 2006; Hammen & Brennan, 2003; Silverman, 1989), an assessment is a necessary prerequisite for developing and initiating effective interventions that can help at-risk children onto healthier pathways (Gambrill, 2005; Herman, 1997; Nicholson & Blanch, 1994; Oyserman, Mowbray, & Zemencuk, 1994; Rutter, 1995).

Determining whether a parent with mental illness poses significant risks to children can be a daunting task. Part of what makes parenting assessments so daunting is the inherent difficulty of predicting future behavior (Grisso & Appelbaum, 1992). Mental illnesses are not uniform entities. They vary in etiology, symptomatology, clinical course, and prognosis (American Psychiatric Association, 2000). These factors can all affect parenting to different degrees (Alpern & Lyons-Ruth, 1993). Parenting, itself, is not a uniform entity. It is a multifaceted role that requires different skills depending on a child's developmental stage and needs (Göpfert, Webster, & Nelki, 2004b; Solomon & George, 1996). In addition, parenting and mental illness can both change over time. Both are profoundly influenced by context—personal, familial, environmental, and cultural (Belsky, 1993; Göpfert et al., 2004b).

During formal assessments, parents are likely to experience high levels of stress and may act differently, knowing that their every behavior is being scrutinized. Some may falsify information or be less than forthright about parenting difficulties, which makes it more challenging to determine whether actual risks and competencies have been evaluated. Others may be understandably upset, angry, or resentful about inquiries into their lives and may withhold important information from assessors.

Children are also under stress, sensing that an assessment is upsetting for their parents and could change their family situation. In this situation, they, too, may withhold critical information about experiences with their parents and how they are faring emotionally and in other areas of their lives. All of these factors may make it difficult to determine parenting risks and strengths.

The time involvement and responsibility demanded by mental health professionals also make assessments daunting. Interviewing parents and children, observing interactions, visiting the home, writing reports, scheduling feedback sessions, and giving court testimony are part and parcel of the involvement required to complete an assessment. How questions about parenting competency and risk are addressed will also have immense consequences for families, contributing to the responsibility of the assessor. For instance, if an assessment reveals that a child is at a high risk for being harmed, the child may be removed from the parent's care. Although this is necessary in some cases, disruptions in care are likely to have long-lasting consequences for the well-being and lives of both parents and children (Bowlby, 1973, 1988).

This book draws on recent literature and on clinical experience to provide an overview of how mental health professionals can approach assessments of parenting in individuals with mental illness. The ideas presented in this book are a personal synthesis of my work on a multidisciplinary parenting assessment team (Jacobsen & Miller, 1998b; Jacobsen, Miller, & Kirkwood, 1997), my clinical work with parents and children, theories of development, and current research findings. The organizing themes come from a combination of attachment theory, ecological theories of child maltreatment, and research on violence risk potential.

Attachment theory provides a rich basis for understanding the centrality of parenting in the lives of most individuals, the bonds of love that bind parent and child to each other, and the reasons why a parent takes care of a child in the particular way he or she does. It emphasizes the parent's own attachment history and the role of the parent's current state of mind toward these experiences as major determinants of parenting (Bowlby, 1988; Lyons-Ruth, Yellin, Melnick, & Atwood; 2005; Solomon & George, 1996). Attachment theory also provides a framework for understanding the child's attachment to his or her caregivers and how these bonds influence the child's ability to explore, the quality of relationships he or she forms with others, and the effects of separation and loss on a child's sense of self and long-term well-being (Bowlby, 1988).

A basic premise of ecological theory is that child neglect and abuse result from a broad range of environmental and familial factors that interact with each other over time (Belsky, 1993; Cicchetti & Toth, 1995; Hill, Fonagy, Safier, & Sargent, 2003; Tolan, Gorman-Smith, & Henry, 2003). In ecological theory, focus is on the role of parental and child characteristics, parent–child interactions, intergenerational and family dynamics, and cultural and societal factors in compromising a parent's ability to nurture and provide adequate care and protection for the child. Ecological theory provides a rich framework for understanding the dynamics of parenting breakdown and for isolating critical factors at the individual, family, cultural, and societal levels that contribute to parenting risk and competency. It also considers the strengths that an individual brings to the parenting role and factors that can ameliorate risk and promote more healthy parenting pathways (Cicchetti & Toth, 1995).

Violence risk potential research provides a powerful framework for understanding when an individual with mental illness who has been violent in the past poses a substantial risk of harming others either now or in the future (Bloom, Webster, Hucker, & De Freitas, 2005; Dolan & Doyle, 2000; Monahan et al., 2000; Steadman et al., 1994). As with ecological theory, this approach views violence risk potential as a complex and multifaceted phenomenon and underscores the importance of assessing a comprehensive array of theory-based risk factors in multiple domains of functioning. Some domains that are considered in an assessment of violence risk potential include a parent's own childhood experiences, and her current disposition (e.g., angry, impulsive, psychopathic), as well as situations that could evoke risk behaviors.

An important part of violence risk potential is its emphasis on the need for a careful examination of the contribution of specific mental illness symptoms (e.g., delusions, hallucinations, violent fantasies to violence), as well as an examination of the course and prognosis of the illness and the individual's responsiveness to interventions (Monahan et al., 2000). This approach underscores that risk is not something static but can change over time and in different contexts (Monahan et al., 2000). Assessing parenting risk, then, always involves an estimation of probabilities, estimating how likely it is that harm will occur now or in the near future.

Current assessments of parenting competency and risk have been shown to have serious methodological flaws (e.g., Blanch, Nicholson, & Purcell, 1994; Jacobsen et al., 1997; Nicholson, Geller, Fisher, & Dion, 1993). Common problems include the use of instruments that measure aspects of a parent's psychological functioning but that are not directly relevant to parenting risk (Azar, Lauretti, & Loding, 1998; Brodzinsky, 1993; Budd & Holdsworth, 1996; Grisso, 2002), a reliance on evidence derived from only a few assessment tools, the observation of a parent in only one context, the use of optimal instead of minimal parenting competency as a standard, a failure to take into account cultural differences in child-rearing practices, the use of instruments that have not been systematically validated on parents with mental disorders (Jacobsen et al., 1997), and a focus on parenting weaknesses and deficits (Ackerson, 2003; Budd, Poindexter, Felix, & Naik-Polan, 2001).

Although a rich body of literature exists that can guide parenting assessments of individuals with mental disorders, this knowledge is neither routinely translated into sound assessment strategies (Budd et al., 2001) nor routinely taught in medical schools, graduate programs, residencies, or internships. Attorneys, judges, and service coordinators rarely receive specialized training in what constitutes a sound parenting assessment. This lack of specialized training, combined with the use of unsound assessment tools, can result in mistakes in decision-making processes (Gambrill, 2005). Such errors are costly and can contribute to serious injuries to or the death of a child, longstanding emotional distress for families, or permanent separations between parents and children. Therefore, using a sound assessment methodology is essential.

Biases about mental illness and its effects on parenting are other important reasons why a book about parenting assessment is needed. Mental illness still constitutes a stigma for many people in society (Burton, 1990; Seeman & Göpfert, 2004). Moreover, in news media and reporting, mental illness is often portrayed as being synonymous with or closely linked to dangerous and irrational behavior (Link & Cullen, 1986; Monahan, 1992). It is not surprising, then, that parents with mental illness are viewed from a pathological perspective (Ackerson, 2003).

Unfortunately, these perceptions contribute to existing fears about the relation between mental illness and parenting and fuel the view that mental illness may be incompatible with good parenting (e.g., Murphy, 1996). Because many parents with mental illness are clearly able to successfully raise their children on their own or with the help of others (Nicholson et al., 1998a), decision making and planning should be based on sound assessments and not on existing biases or fears about mental illness.

Finally, sound assessments are essential because they form the basis for implementing meaningful interventions that can make a difference for vulnerable parents and their children (Gambrill, 2005; Jordan & Franklin, 2003; Nicholson & Blanch, 1994; Oyserman et al., 1994).

The guidelines outlined in this book are designed to enable clinicians to provide a comprehensive assessment of parenting competency and risk. The assessment methodology outlined in this book emphasizes the need to observe parenting directly, to gather information on various facets of parenting (e.g., maternal attitudes, cognitive understanding of development, internal representations of children), to rely on different measures and sources of information, and to elucidate how different contexts (e.g., family support, environmental factors, mental illness) may impede or facilitate a parent's ability to care for children. A review of records and the use of critical thinking are essential parts of this approach (Gambrill, 2005; Jacobsen et al., 1997).

This book emphasizes that the process of assessment involves comparing data from different sources and different points in time in order to identify patterns that will aid in drawing conclusions about parenting competency and risk (Azar et al., 1998; Budd et al., 2001; Gambrill, 2005; Lincoln & Guba, 1985; Strauss & Corbin, 1998). It also emphasizes the need to assess a parent's strengths and competencies and to examine how well a mother can meet the unique needs of each of her children (Ackerson, 2003). Clinical expertise is used while data from various sources are sorted through and integrated, and careful attention is given to ethical issues, including informed consent, transparency of practices, and an honest brokering of knowledge and uncertainties (Gambrill, 2006). Finally, the book underscores the need for an organized research-informed framework to help clinicians conduct parenting assessments if and when they are needed.

The book is organized into eight substantive chapters. Chapter 2 lays the groundwork for the assessment by providing an overview of major types of mental illness and how different mental illness symptoms affect parenting. The next chapters of the book are devoted to the assessment itself. Chapters 3 and 4 provide an overview of assessment guidelines and the assessment process. Chapters 5–8 detail the components of the individual domains of the assessment. These include assessing a mother's caregiving capabilities; looking at psychiatric environmental and familial factors that may have an impact on parenting; and determining children's well-being, development, and needs. The final chapter, Chapter 9, includes a narrative of an adult who, during her childhood, experienced her mother's mental illness. That chapter gives firsthand descriptions of some of the experiences and themes that assessors are likely to encounter in children.

This book includes two appendices. The first provides a list of various tools that might be useful in assessing parenting competency and risk. The second appendix lists books and resources on the topics of mental illness, parenting, and assessment that will aid clinicians in their learning endeavor. Two chapters in the book (7 and 9) were written by social workers: a colleague, and a student of mine. Both have expertise in mental illness and parenting.

The larger aim of the book is to improve decision making for individuals with mental illness who struggle in the parenting role by grounding assessments in empirical research, through sound clinical practice, and by linking assessments to interventions that can make a difference for parents and children alike (e.g., Nicholson, Biebel, Hinden, Henry, & Stier, 2001).

A few points need to be addressed at the outset. First, this book draws on current knowledge and clinical experience to illustrate how mental health professionals can assess parenting competency and risk in primary caregivers. Although the primary caregiver can be the father (Ackerson, 2003; Nicholson, Nason, Calebresi, & Yando, 1999), women with mental illness are far more likely than men to be involved in child care (Hatfield, Webster, & Mohamad, 1997; Seeman & Göpfert, 2004). For this reason, the book's main focus is on women as parents.

Second, the book is primarily written for mental health professionals; that is, the book is designed for clinicians who have experience working with families and parents with mental illness or who are training to acquire this experience. These individuals include mental health professionals with backgrounds in psychiatry, social work, psychology, nursing, and counseling. However, components of these guidelines may also be useful for child welfare professionals, service coordinators, attorneys, judges, and home visitors seeking to make sound decisions for individuals with mental illness and their families.

A basic premise underlying the guidelines presented in this book is that the clinician's assessment skills will be grounded in a solid clinical background and a working knowledge of mental disorders, parenting, and child development. The parenting capabilities and risks that clinicians will encounter in their work will widely vary in level and strength. The variability is even greater when the full course of parenting is considered. Risk can be encountered during pregnancy, in the postpartum period, and at later periods in the parenting cycle. For this reason, I place less emphasis on recommending one specific assessment format, arguing instead for a sound approach to assessments and one that is closely informed by knowledge of mental illness, parenting, and child development.

Third, because the book examines how parenting capability and risk can be assessed in individuals with mental illness, some comment should be made at the outset about how mental illness is defined. In this book, mental illness is seen as being synonymous with psychiatric disorder. An individual who is diagnosed with a psychiatric disorder experiences clinically significant distress or impairment in social, occupational, and other important functional areas. He or she also evidences a pattern of symptoms that meet criteria for a specific psychiatric disorder in the *Diagnostic and Statistical Manual of Mental Disorders, Fourth Edition, Text Revision* (*DSM-IV-TR*; American Psychiatric Association, 2000), the standard manual that is used for diagnosing mental disorders in the United States.

Mental illness symptoms vary greatly in individuals—even those with the same disorder—ranging on a continuum from mild to severe. Moreover, symptoms can wax and wane over time. Manifestations of mental illness can also vary with age, gender, race, and culture. This book focuses on parenting in individuals who have a clinical disorder (i.e., a diagnosable mental illness in the *DSM-IV-TR* or other comparable manuals). Because parenting is almost always affected to some degree when the individual's illness is chronic and severe, this book gives more focus to disorders that are chronic and severe.

Fourth, although this book is designed to cover a broad range of circumstances in which a parenting assessment may be needed, parenting assessments are only necessary in certain situations. As I emphasize again and again, many parents with mental illness are capable of safely raising their children either alone or with the help of others. At the same time, clear circumstances may indicate when an assessment may be necessary to guide decision-making and to plan effective parenting rehabilitation. A parenting assessment is needed if there is evidence or strong suspicion that a child is being neglected or abused, if substantial risks are posed to the well-being and development of a child, and if a child has been placed in state custody and questions about future parenting competency must be addressed. Assessments may also be immensely useful in determining what types of intervention will best help to address parenting that has been compromised in individuals with psychiatric disorders. This book is designed to help mental health professionals face these circumstances.

2

Mental Illness

Types and Effects on Parenting

Michelle was 29 years old when she first experienced serious psychiatric symptoms. She began to feel restless and had difficulty sleeping. Her thoughts raced, and, at times, she felt elated. Until her symptoms emerged, Michelle had done well in raising her two young children, Tony and Mae. But one night when it was bitter cold outside, Michelle left the house and started walking. She carried Tony, age 2 months, in a thin blanket. Mae, age 6 years, wore a summer sweater and walked resolutely beside her mother. When a bystander approached Michelle, Michelle could not say where she and her children were headed.

Studies underscore that about one third of women in the United States and one fifth of men show evidence of psychiatric disorder (Nicholson, Biebel, Hinden, Henry, & Stier, 2001). The majority of these individuals are parents. Although many parents with mental illness are able to care for their children either on their own or with support (Ritscher, Coursey, & Farrell, 1997), others, such as Michelle, struggle in the parenting role. In some instances, their psychiatric symptoms can interfere with judgment, behavior, feelings, or energy to the point that they seriously compromise their ability to discipline children, to establish appropriate boundaries, and to provide for their children's basic needs and safety (Ackerson, 2003).

For mothers whose illness is persistent and severe, risk for serious parenting problems is especially high (Grunbaum & Gammeltoft, 1993). Studies estimate that as many as 60 to 80% of women with severe mental illness may relinquish or lose custody of their children at some point in their lives (Nicholson et al., 2001). In some cases, relatives or friends may care for children during periods in which a mother needs to be hospitalized due to illness exacerbations.

Although custody loss can occur at any time in the parenting span, some evidence suggests that it may occur more frequently after birth (Kumar, Marks, Platz, & Yoshida, 1995) or in the early years of parenting (Ruppert &

Bagedahl-Strindlund, 2001), probably because women are at an especially high risk for developing a psychiatric disorder or for experiencing illness exacerbations in these periods (Cohen, Sichel, Robertson, Heckscher, & Rosenbaum, 1995).

For cases in which the parenting pathway is uncertain, an assessment may be useful, and even essential, both for establishing whether the mother's illness symptoms pose significant risks to her parenting and to her children's well-being and for determining what interventions or treatment regimens may help the family onto a healthier pathway.

A best-practices approach to the assessment of parenting requires assessors to draw on scientific knowledge about parenting in individuals with mental illness. They should have a solid knowledge of different mental disorders and an understanding of how different mental illness symptoms can contribute to parenting risk and impact children's development. Assessors will also need to understand mothers' perspectives and needs. Depending on the specific circumstances of the family, this information is then flexibly used in an assessment and is considered in designing interventions to address parents' needs.

This chapter provides an overview of these topics. It first focuses on the perspectives and needs of parents with mental illness, underscoring the centrality of the parenting role in their lives. Major types of psychiatric disorders, including schizophrenia, bipolar disorder, depression, anxiety disorders, personality disorders, and the abuse of substances are then described. After this, I examine how various psychiatric symptoms characteristic of these disorders can affect parenting and contribute to parenting risk.

PERSPECTIVES AND THEMES

Parenting is a central life role for mothers with mental illness (Apfel & Handel, 1993; Nicholson, Sweeney, & Geller, 1998b). Mothers with mental illness consistently underscore that parenting gives them a purpose in life, a sense of identity, love, and long-term support as their children grow up (Chernomas, Clarke, & Chisholm, 2000). As one mother noted, "Motherhood is a wonderful, fulfilling experience, one that women with a mental illness have every right to experience and enjoy" (Fox, 1999, p. 194).

Although parenting is a central life role, mothers with mental illness often face formidable challenges as they struggle to fill dual roles (Ackerson, 2003; Nicholson et al., 1998b). They must look after their own emotional needs and manage an illness that causes impairment in social functioning and judgment, while simultaneously meeting the stresses of parenting and the needs of their children as they change and grow.

A special challenge that many mothers with mental illness face is that although they have a strong desire to be good mothers, the stress of parenting can exacerbate their symptoms. Many mothers in this situation need help learning how to recognize their symptoms and manage their illness while also leaning effective parenting techniques. Special interventions that address the interaction between the demands and stress of being a parent and the symptoms of their particular illness are also needed.

Researchers who have interviewed mothers to obtain their perspectives on what it is like to be a parent while living with mental illness find several common themes. Many mothers with mental illness often judge themselves too harshly as parents (Nicholson et al., 1998b). They may view their children's behavior through the lens of their illness and worry that their children's behavior indicates that the children are developing emotional disturbance themselves (Nicholson et al., 1998b). Many mothers with mental illness understand that their parenting becomes impaired when they relapse (Diaz-Caneja & Johnson, 2004). Others may have difficulties in acknowledging that they have a mental illness or that it can negatively impact parenting.

Many individuals with mental illness are wary of psychotropic medication. Some of this wariness is likely due to the side effects of medication, although some mothers believe that medication may have a negative impact on parenting. Indeed, high doses of psychotropic medication can contribute to tiredness or other side effects that can make it difficult for a mother to be fully available to respond to her children's cues. For some mothers, a wariness of taking psychotropic medication may begin during pregnancy and may be linked to the belief that by not taking medication, they can protect their unborn babies from harm (Nicholson et al., 1998b).

Clinicians who work with mothers with mental illness are likely to encounter themes of stigma, loneliness, loss, grief, and isolation (Apfel & Handel, 1993), themes that are often revisited in different guises with each new assessment.

Because of the stigma associated with mental illness, many mothers may be reluctant to talk about their illness and symptoms with mental health professionals or may be hesitant to seek help for their parenting. As one mother said, "I don't tell. I just find that . . . they don't understand . . . they think they're going to be murdered by you, so I don't like to mention anything" (Chernomas et al., 2000, p. 1518). Another mother noted, "It is quite hard to ask for help when you need it because everybody thinks, 'Oh she's a bad mother, she can't do this' " (Diaz-Caneja & Johnson, 2004, p. 476). Talking openly about parenting difficulties can also have consequences. Children may be removed from a mother's care if a mother reveals neglectful or abusive actions.

Loneliness and isolation are other themes that characterize the lives of many mothers with mental illness. Many describe themselves as feeling invisible and as having a tenuous sense of self. Some of the invisibleness may be linked to fears of talking about themselves and how others will perceive them. Loss and grief are other common experiences in the lives of mothers with major mental illness. Temporary or permanent custody loss leads to drastic changes in family life and introduces immense stress in both a mother's life and in the lives of her children. Losing custody is extremely painful and traumatic for all mothers. One mother noted the following:

> In the past when I was in hospital I would have a picture of my daughter and work towards getting well. . . . This time around I wouldn't be going back to full-time parenting, and I was in hospital a long time. . . . I wasn't getting my daughter back. In fact, I felt destitute, like I'd lost everything in the world. (Diaz-Caneja & Johnson, 2000, p. 477)

When parental rights are terminated, the pain of loss can persist indefinitely and haunt a mother. One woman stayed in the same home for more than 20 years in case her child came to locate her (Chernomas et al., 2000). Another mother carried a ragged photograph of her baby in her wallet for years. When the mother was hospitalized for postpartum psychosis 20 years prior, she gave up her baby for adoption. Mothers who have lost custody of their child often experience an ongoing fear that they may lose custody again (Diaz-Caneja & Johnson, 2004; Venkataraman, 2005).

The aforementioned perspectives and themes provide an essential lens for understanding how mothers may respond to a parenting assessment. Assessments are likely to heighten parents' anxiety and make them feel vulnerable and powerless. Talking about their illness and its effects on their children can be difficult due to the stigma of the illness and to a perceived sense of rejection.

Inquiring into a mother's feelings about her children and her role as parent and paying attention to her needs and her viewpoints on what might help—including what types of services may be of use to her as a parent—are important tasks for clinicians. A working alliance is likely to be more easily established if clinicians are interested in a mother's experiences and views. In turn, a mother is likely to be more open about her difficulties as a parent as well as be more receptive to feedback and treatment if her position is understood and considered by clinicians in the assessment and feedback process.

MENTAL ILLNESS AND PARENTING

It is important to keep in mind that many mothers with mental illness are able to adequately care for their children (Jacobsen & Miller, 1998a; Oates, 1997; Reder, McClure, & Jolley, 2000). In such cases, a mother is likely to be compliant with and responsive to treatment, have good coping skills, and have good insight into her illness (Mullick, Miller, & Jacobsen, 2001). In addition, the mother is likely to be able to establish and maintain good supportive relationships with others who help her, both individually and in a parenting role. At the same time, a psychiatric illness can increase parenting risk, especially if the illness symptoms are chronic and severe.

The *DSM-IV-TR* presents the criteria for determining whether an individual has a diagnosable mental illness and, if so, what type of mental disorder he or she has. Individuals who are diagnosed with a mental illness evidence a pattern of symptoms that meet criteria for a specific psychiatric disorder, and they also experience clinically significant distress or impairment in social, occupational, and other important functional areas. The following sections describe psychiatric disorders that clinicians are likely to encounter in assessments and discuss various psychiatric symptoms that can affect parenting.

Schizophrenia

Schizophrenia is characterized by episodic and sometimes ongoing disturbances of thought, perception, speech, and affect (American Psychiatric Association, 2000). An individual with schizophrenia has two types of symptoms: negative and positive. Negative symptoms involve a diminution or loss of functioning, such as blunted affect, apathy, self-neglect, loss of motivation, difficulty with abstract thinking, and social withdrawal. Positive symptoms involve an excess or distortion of normal functions and include psychotic symptoms such as hallucinatory behavior, conceptual disorganization, and delusions.

Schizophrenia can result in the deterioration of an individual's work, social, and self-care functioning and in difficulties in establishing long-term relationships with the opposite sex, although women with schizophrenia usually have better social functioning than men (Seeman, 2006).

The course and symptoms of schizophrenia can also make it difficult for mothers to provide consistent long-term care for their children (Miller, 1997), although parenting skills vary widely within individuals with this diagnosis. Rates of custody loss are high in mothers with schizophrenia and exceed those of mothers with depression or bipolar disorder (Miller & Finnerty, 1996). Many mothers with schizophrenia may care for their children off and on during infancy, childhood, and adolescence, relinquishing their children to the care of a spouse, relatives, or friends when they are hospitalized or experience illness exacerbations (Caton, Cournos, Felix, & Wyatt, 1998).

The postpartum period is a time of particularly high risk for acute exacerbations of schizophrenia (McNeil, Persson-Blennow, Binett, Harty, & Karyd, 1988). Some mothers who are hospitalized for psychoses in the postpartum period develop aberrant attitudes about childbirth and about their infant. For example, they may believe the birth did not occur or that the baby is defective or even dead (Stewart, 1984). Risk of harm is particularly high if the baby becomes part of the mother's delusions and if relatives are not available to help the mother after she is released from the hospital (Appleby & Dickens, 1993).

For some mothers with psychotic symptoms, parenting behavior can become unpredictable, ranging from intrusive to uninvolved (Abernathy & Grunebaum, 1972). If a mother experiences paranoia, she may limit her child's contact with others outside the family, reducing potential support and the child's ability to check reality.

Whereas positive symptoms of schizophrenia (hallucinations and delusions) may greatly impair parenting, negative symptoms (emotional withdrawal, blunted affect) can reduce a mother's ability to convey affect, and may impede her ability to engage in mutual interchanges with her child (Persson-Blennow, Binett, & McNeil, 1988). Cognitive deficits and problems in forming coherent thoughts, other negative symptoms of schizophrenia, can contribute to a mother misinterpreting and overreacting to her child's behavior.

Some mothers with overt psychotic symptoms may include a child in their delusions. This may result in a *folie à deux*—a shared psychotic disorder—a condition whereby a child comes to accept the veracity of her mother's delusions (Anthony, 1971). In one case, a child, age 8 years, shared her mother's delusion that intergalactic rays were penetrating them. The child was afraid to go outside for fear that a neighbor would rape her. A *folie à deux* is more frequent when the mother and child have a highly dependent relationship and are socially isolated.

Mothers with overt psychotic behavior may engage in bizarre behavior and may violate social norms. This behavior can be painful and troubling for older children who may feel embarrassed or ashamed of their mother's behavior and of their own feelings about her. Holley (Holley & Holley, 1997) vividly described such feelings in her autobiography. Her mother was diagnosed with schizophrenia when Holley was a young child:

> Mama was wearing a wrinkled dress . . . mis-buttoned so that you could see her bra. She had slipped into a pair of dingy old house slippers, the heels bent down beneath her feet. She occasionally looked to the side as if carrying on a conversation with an invisible companion . . . I wanted to tear my hair out, kick down the garage, do something to gouge out the pain and anger and guilt I felt. (p. 173)

Women with positive symptoms of schizophrenia may have more positive treatment outcomes than mothers with marked negative symptoms (Davies, McIvor, & Kumar, 1995). Consistent, long-term use of antipsychotic medication can significantly decrease the frequency and severity of active psychotic symptoms and can improve a mother's ability to parent (Altshuler & Kiriakos, 2006). However, when medication is too sedating, it can interfere with a mother's ability to monitor her children's whereabouts and to remain responsive to their needs.

Depression

The most common psychiatric disorder in the *DSM-IV-TR* is major depression. Ten to twenty percent of new mothers develop clinical depression after giving birth to their babies. The rates double in samples of low-income mothers and in mothers who give birth to their baby during adolescence.

Individuals who are diagnosed with clinical depression feel more than just sad or blue. They experience one or more major depressive episodes. According to the *DSM-IV-TR* (American Psychiatric Association, 2000), the symptoms of a major depressive episode include anhedonia—the inability to experience pleasure from normally pleasurable life events nearly all of the time, decreased energy, and chronic sadness or depression. In addition, individuals experience changes in eating or sleeping, feel helpless or hopeless, have problems with concentration, and are socially withdrawn. Individuals who experience recurring episodes of clinical depression have a psychiatric disability that can impair their ability to function socially, at work, and as a parent. Postpartum depression involves the same symptoms as those that occur with clinical depression at other points in life. The symptoms, however, occur within 6 months after a woman has given birth to her child.

Postpartum depression should not be confused with the postpartum blues, which is a normal experience that many women go through after giving birth to a baby. Between 26% and 85% of women experience the blues in the postpartum period (O'Hara, Zekoski, Philipps, & Wright, 1990). The blues typically occur within the first 10 days after birth. Women who develop the blues experience transient feelings of depressed mood, increased crying spells, irritability, and a sense of unreality in the immediate postpartum period (Chaudron, 2003).

Mothers with postpartum depression may be emotionally unavailable and have difficulties in responding to their infant's cues (Cohn, Campbell, Matias, & Hopkins, 1990; Martins & Gaffan, 2000). Others may be intrusive or display hostile affect toward their infants. If a mother with postpartum depression has a tentative hold on reality, she may be at an especially high risk for harming her baby (Chandra, Venkatasubramanian, & Thomas, 2002). In such cases, inpatient hospitalization may be essential to help decrease her depressive symptoms.

Recognizing the risk factors for postpartum depression may avert unfortunate outcomes. Important risk factors include the following: a previous history of major depression, a family history of mood disorder, marital discord, poor support, and several stressful life events in the year prior to delivery (O'Hara, 1986).

Ongoing, untreated depression can contribute to a mother developing distorted expectations of and perceptions about her children. A severely depressed mother may lower expectations for her child's achievements (Whiffen & Gotlib, 1989). In interacting with her child, a mother who is depressed may show more negative behavior, less engagement, and higher levels of criticism (Tarullo, DeMulder, Ronsaville, Brown, & Radke-Yarrow, 1995). She may also have difficulty tolerating the child's own sadness and, as a result, may view the child as burdensome. Children, in turn, may internalize and accept the views their mothers have of them, becoming overly critical of themselves and developing a depressive mindset.

When a depressed mother is suicidal, issues of safety toward her children loom large. A mother may plan to kill herself and her children to avoid abandoning them. One mother, for instance, parked her car on the train tracks with her children when she was severely depressed. Her oldest son convinced her to move off of the tracks at the last minute, thus averting tragedy. Children who witness or experience a maternal suicide or suicide attempts are at a high risk for developing long-term emotional problems (Bowlby, 1988).

Bipolar Disorder

In bipolar disorder, a mother alternately experiences depression and mania. In the depressed phase, a mother may experience a loss of interest or pleasure, depressed mood, diminished ability to think or concentrate, and disturbances in body weight and sleep. In the manic phase of bipolar disorder, she may experience expansive, elevated, or irritable moods; grandiosity; hyperactivity; decreased sleep; pressured speech; excessive involvement in pleasurable activities that have a high potential for painful consequences (e.g., unrestrained buying sprees); or a flight of ideas (American Psychiatric Association, 2000).

Bipolar disorder is considered a chronic mental disorder, and in many cases it results in psychiatric disability and difficulties in social and occupational functioning. Nonetheless, many people with bipolar disorder are able to hold jobs, engage in social relationships, and raise children, although their ability to function in these roles can be compromised when they experience an episode of major depression or mania. A large number of individuals with bipolar disorder do not regain full occupational and social functioning even though their illness is in remission (MacQueen, Young, & Joffe, 2001).

Although postpartum psychosis is rare and affects only 1 or 2 women of 100, it occurs much more frequently in women with bipolar disorder (Viguera, Cohen, Baldessarini, & Nonacs, 2002). Postpartum psychosis poses a high immediate risk to infants (Finnerty, Levin, & Miller, 1996; Sneddon, Kerry, & Bant, 1981) but not necessarily long-term risk if treatment is effective (Persson-Blennow et al., 1988). For example, one mother with postpartum mania who threatened to kill her newborn had not been on any mood-stabilizing medication during pregnancy. Her psychosis necessitated a separation from the infant, which was highly distressing to the mother. Risk of harm decreased after she began taking her medication regularly and after it was established that she was responsive to the medication.

The lack of judgment, impulsive behavior, and unstable lifestyles that characterize the behaviors of many mothers with untreated bipolar mood disorder can contribute to insensitive and unpredictable maternal behavior. During a manic phase of her illness, one mother, for instance, pulled her daughter's leg roughly, causing a spiral fracture. The mother was unaware of this and could hardly believe that it had happened. Mothers with bipolar disorder may show excessive anger in interacting with their children, a lack of leadership, and unclear communication (Radke-Yarrow, Nottelmann, Belmont, & Welsh, 1993).

A study comparing mothers with bipolar disorder to well mothers found that mothers with bipolar disorder were less engaged, less affectionate, and more prone to show negative and downcast affect when playing with their children (DeMulder & Radke-Yarrow, 1991). Two thirds of the children who had mothers with bipolar disorder showed insecure attachment quality in a standard observation as compared with 42% of the children with well mothers. A large proportion of index children showed characteristic features of disorganized attachment, an at-risk attachment pattern that has been linked to later emotional, behavioral, and psychiatric difficulties in children (Lyons-Ruth & Jacobvitz, 1999).

Posttraumatic Conditions

Individuals who are exposed to a life-threatening event or a threat of serious injury may develop a severe anxiety disorder in response to their trauma. Posttraumatic symptoms are grouped in three categories: re-experiencing the event, numbing and an avoidance of stimuli associated with the trauma, and increased arousal. Re-experiencing often takes the form of recurring and intrusive images and thoughts, distressing dreams or nightmares, flashbacks, and other feelings as if the trauma were recurring. Avoidance behaviors may be related to avoiding feelings or thoughts about the trauma, as well as avoiding people, places, and activities. Arousal symptoms include irritability and hypervigilant behavior as well as physical symptoms (American Psychiatric Association, 2000).

Dissociative Identity Disorder (DID) is another posttraumatic condition that results from life-threatening events. It reflects a failure to integrate various aspects of memory, identity, and consciousness. An individual experiences different personality states that have a distinct personal history, identity, self-image, and name. Although a primary identity usually carries the individual's name, more aggressive identities may interrupt activities or place the individual and others in difficult situations (American Psychiatric Association, 2000).

Mothers with posttraumatic conditions are often at a heightened risk for abusing their own children. Kluft (1987) studied the parenting skills of 75 mothers with DID. Sixteen percent had harmed their children physically, had sexually abused them, or had failed to protect them from harm. Another 45% had fewer, but still significant, difficulties in responsibly caring for their children. Most mothers in the study were highly distressed by their parenting problems.

Although severe posttraumatic stress disorder (PTSD) can place a mother at risk for child maltreatment, risk of abuse is substantially decreased if a mother has been able to work through the sequelae of childhood traumas in therapy. However, working through the trauma experiences may initially contribute to more difficulties in parenting:

Loretta had been sexually abused in childhood by a neighbor. She didn't tell anyone about the abuse because the man who abused her had threatened to harm her mother and sister if she told. Because her constant flashbacks, nightmares, and hypervigilance were affecting how she responded to her children's distress, Loretta sought out a therapist for help. As she began to trust the therapist enough to reveal the abuse to her, Loretta's parenting skills plummeted. She had particular difficulties in responding to her children's distress. As she worked through her trauma, however, Loretta became more able to recognize her children's distress. Her comfort level in holding her children also improved as therapy progressed.

A mother with DID may have major attentional lapses, or "blackout" periods, during which time she may remember nothing, leave home, and/or abandon her children. Suicide attempts and psychiatric hospitalizations, also common in mothers with DID, can profoundly affect a mother's ability to attend to her children's needs (Benjamin, Benjamin, & Rind, 1996). Risk of child maltreatment is increased in mothers who experience their children as abusers and who view themselves as a child (Lyons-Ruth & Jacobvitz, 1999).

One mother who saw her child as an abuser, for instance, screamed and fell to the floor. She then begged the child not to harm her. The child, a 5-year-old boy, was confused and upset by his mother's behavior.

Anxiety Disorders

Anxiety is an important physiological response that is shown by individuals in dangerous situations. It prepares an individual to evade or confront threats. If the mechanisms that regulate anxiety break down, the individual experiences excessive anxiety. Symptoms of anxiety include shortness of breath, rapid heart rate, trembling, restlessness, muscle tension, lightheadedness, or dizziness.

Obsessive-compulsive disorder (OCD), one type of anxiety disorder, is characterized by recurring and intrusive thoughts or images (obsessions) and repetitive behaviors or mental acts (compulsions) that an individual feels compelled to perform in response to the obsession. Some compulsive behaviors, such as excessive hand washing, are readily observable. Yet others, such as counting or checking, are more internal. Obsessive and compulsive behaviors are time consuming and cause significant functional impairment and personal distress. Adults with OCD are aware that their behavior is abnormal, but they feel as if they have little or no control over their thoughts and behaviors.

Anxiety disorders can affect parenting in many ways. A parent with OCD, for instance, may demand too much from his or her child and become obsessive about how a child should complete a task. The self-doubting that characterizes individuals with this disorder can be emotionally burdensome and contribute to a young child doubting his or her abilities. Parents with anxiety disorders may become highly distressed or anxious when their children are away or engaged in routine activities. Children in turn may become anxious when they are alone or if they are separated from their parents.

Personality Disorders

A personality disorder involves an "enduring pattern of inner experience and behavior that deviates markedly from the expectations of the individual's culture and is manifested in at least two of the following areas: cognition, affectivity, interpersonal functioning, or impulse control" (American Psychiatric Association, 2000, p. 686). This pattern of behavior or inner experience is pervasive across situations, is inflexible, and leads to impairment in various areas of functioning.

The following behaviors that are characteristic of personality disorder can greatly interfere with parenting (Adshead, Falkov, & Göpfert, 2004): a lack of empathy, violence to self and others, impulsive behavior, and poor affect control. Mothers with personality disorders have serious difficulties with their social and occupational functioning. These problems can contribute to a mother having difficulties in sustaining a safe, predictable environment.

Many parents with personality disorders are victims of childhood abuse and neglect (Flynn, Matthews, & Hollins, 2002). During the years of early childhood and adolescence, their own needs for protection and love were not adequately met. Individuals with this disorder have coped by strongly avoiding having to think about their caregiver's wish to harm them (Schachnow et al., 1997). This avoidance may leave them vulnerable in intimate relationships, including those with their children in which they may fail to adequately register danger. In addition, they may have difficulties in tolerating their children's anger or distress and/or may place their child in a parental role. As seen in the next vignette, such individuals may also have difficulties in maintaining clear interpersonal boundaries (Ostler & Haight, n.d.) and may establish relationships with their children that are based on unhealthy past relationships rather than on current experiences (Bowlby, 1988).

Janie, a mother with a personality disorder, was impulsive and exhibited emotional instability. When her 2-year-old child, Jack, cried, Janie could not tolerate his emotions and taunted him by placing him in a window sill and threatening to leave. Later, she told Jack that he had hurt her and didn't love her enough. Janie's emotional instability contributed to high levels of insecurity in Jack and to difficulties he had in soothing himself. Janie's difficulties in tolerating her son's feelings appeared to be closely linked to her own mother's difficulties in tolerating Janie's feelings when Janie was a child.

Parents with a personality disorder may show hostile behavior toward their children and resort to impulsive acts of discipline rather than try to intervene verbally with their children. Researchers in one study found that depressed mothers who had an underlying personality disorder were more critical of, irritable toward, and psychologically unavailable to their children than depressed mothers without a personality disorder (DeMulder, Tarulla, Klimes-Dougan, Free, & Radke-Yarrow, 1995).

A mother with a personality disorder may have marked difficulties in taking her child's perspective and in understanding her child's unique developmental needs (Norton & Dolan, 1996). For example, one mother celebrated her own birthday by placing a birthday cake in her child's bed. She told the clinician that she also gave the child, a one-year-old girl, a knife so that the girl could cut the cake herself. The lack of flexibility that characterizes personality disorders may make it difficult for a mother to change her parenting skills to adapt to a child's developmental stage and needs. For example, one mother with a personality disorder refused to believe that her infant was hungry, even though her therapist and family repeatedly pointed out that he was crying and could not eat the mashed carrots the mother had put in his bottle. In this case, the mother's rigid way of thinking made it difficult for her to accept feedback and to adapt her parenting to meet her young infant's needs.

Studies have documented small associations between child maltreatment and two personality disorder subtypes: borderline and antisocial personality disorder (Dinwiddie & Bucholz, 1993; Stanley & Penhale, 1999). Whereas individuals with borderline personality disorder show instability of interpersonal relationships, self-image, and feelings, individuals with antisocial personality disorder show a pattern of disregard for and violation of the rights of others (American Psychiatric Association, 2000). Parenting outcomes may be particularly poor for mothers with antisocial personality disorder (Robins, 1966). Change can occur for individuals with this diagnosis, but it usually takes considerable time to engage the parent in the treatment process that they may perceive as threatening (Ryle & Kerr, 2002).

Substance Use Disorders

Substance use disorders include both substance dependence and substance abuse (American Psychiatric Association, 2000). An individual who is dependent on a substance continues to use the substance in a compulsive manner despite significant problems related to the substance. He or she also shows evidence of tolerance—meaning the need for increased amounts of the substance to achieve intoxication—and withdrawal symptoms if the substance is not available. An individual who abuses substances, by contrast, experiences the harmful consequences of repeated use of the substance but does not show evidence of tolerance or withdrawal symptoms. A pattern of compulsive use is also absent in substance abuse disorder (American Psychiatric Association, 2000). Often, other psychiatric problems coexist with substance use or dependence, including depression, PTSD, or a personality disorder (Hans, 1999; Triffleman, Marmar, Delucchi, & Ronfeldt, 1995).

Many mothers with addictions have difficulty maintaining stable relationships with other adults (Luthar & Walsh, 1995). This lack of social support, combined with the ongoing need to sustain an addiction, may make it difficult for a mother to provide a daily structure for her child (Greif & Drechsler, 1993). As it is expensive to maintain an addiction, a mother may turn to theft, fraud, drug dealing, abusive partners, or prostitution as sources of income. A mother in this situation may grossly neglect her child's basic needs and/or fail to protect him or her from harmful situations.

Angie, a mother with a cocaine addiction, left her 3-month-old baby in an unlocked car at night as she went to purchase drugs. She returned several hours later. Hearing the baby's cries, neighbors had alerted the police. When Angie returned to the car, she was arrested. Lisa, her baby, had already been taken into custody.

Addiction disorders can have a profound effect on a family's lifestyle. A mother may lose her job, her partner, her home, and/or her health. Many mothers with substance use problems become involved with Child Protective Services and may lose custody of their children (Leventhal, Forsyth, Qi, Johnson, Schroeder, & Votto, 1997). If the child remains with the mother, she may pressure the child to hide her drug use from others (Baker & Carson, 1999; Klee, 1998). In some cases, the child may be asked to buy drugs to support the parent's habit. Children in this situation may be left alone for days at a time (Hans, 2004). In addition, mothers who abuse substances may fail to protect their children from sexual abuse by partners or others in the household.

Because intoxication impairs impulse control, mothers who abuse substances are at an increased risk for abusing their children physically (Besinger, Garland, Litrownik, & Landsverk, 1999; Leventhal et al., 1997). Researchers in one study of hospital and emergency-room evaluations of injuries secondary to abuse found that children who were physically abused were far more likely than other children to have a parent with a cocaine addiction (Wasserman & Leventhal, 1993). These problems are compounded if a mother has a dual diagnosis, such as substance abuse and depression or PTSD.

Mothers who abuse substances have been shown to be less responsive and less positive in their interactions with infants and toddlers than mothers without these problems (Leventhal et al., 1997). They experience higher parenting stress (Schuler, Nair, Black, & Kettinger, 2000), know less about child development, are more verbally abusive toward their children, and perceive that they have little control over their children's behavior (Kaltenbach & Finnegan, 1987). Their children, in turn, are more likely to develop an insecure attachment in infancy (Rodning, Beckwith, & Howard, 1989). In later development, children of parents who abuse substances are also at increased risk for developing anxiety, depressive, conduct, and substance disorders (Merikangas, Dierker, & Szatmari, 1998).

CONCLUDING REMARKS

An assessment of parenting is based on a working knowledge of mental disorders and a grasp on how different mental illness symptoms affect parenting. It is just as essential for mental health professionals to understand the perspectives and needs of mothers with mental illness—how they have been affected by their illness, how they perceive and understand their symptoms, how they feel about parenting and about their children, what they would like to change, and what they feel will help them and their families. Understanding parents' perspectives and needs helps in gaining their willingness to participate in an assessment; it also lays the groundwork so that a clinician can frame interventions in a way that is accessible and meaningful for parents and their families.

3

Guidelines for Assessment

How one approaches an assessment is as important as what is assessed (Pawl & St. John, 1998). *How* tells about processes that matter in an assessment—how a relationship with a parent is established, how the assessment is conducted, and how questions about risk and competency are formulated and communicated to others.

How also determines, to a large degree, what a parent's experiences with mental health professionals will be like. If the *how* of an assessment goes right, a clinician will obtain rich clinical information that will allow him or her to draw sound conclusions about risk and competency. If the *how* of an assessment goes right, it will also increase the likelihood that a parent and other family members will be receptive to feedback and be more willing to consider and engage in recommended services.

This chapter addresses the issue of *how* by providing an orientation to guidelines that underlie a sound assessment of parenting competency. The guidelines outlined in this chapter hold true across settings, individuals, families, and the roles of assessing mental health professionals. Nonetheless, the way the guidelines are implemented may vary depending on the unique questions raised by each individual, on the service setting, and on the disciplines and characteristics of the assessor.

SENSITIVELY APPROACHING INDIVIDUALS

The most important action that a clinician can take in any assessment is to approach each individual and family with sensitivity. Sensitivity implies that the clinician is aware of and interested in listening to and understanding the specific idiosyncrasies of someone else (Lieberman, 1990). It includes learning about individuals' views, experiences, and specific visions for themselves and their family, their background and culture, and the meanings they attach to specific words, behaviors, and experiences (Carlson & Harwood, 1999).

Understanding the specific idiosyncrasies of another individual starts by showing genuine interest in the individual's life circumstances and experiences. This interest is accompanied by respect and by the assessor being responsive to individual and family communications (Barrera, 2003). It also includes gaining an understanding of cultural factors (mental illness, gender, ethnicity, and so forth) that influence how the individual perceives and views the world in the particular way that he or she does.

Clinicians can neither have knowledge about all cultures nor be familiar with all of the numerous variations in practices, speech, and beliefs within even one culture. But they should not be afraid to learn about different backgrounds, beliefs, and practices. To do this, clinicians need to cultivate an attitude of openness to find out what they don't know about a parent's background and history. The clinicians should ask parents and other family members to teach them about their personal history, experiences, culture, and belief systems. The clinician should listen carefully to each individual in the family, suspend judgment, and reflect on what is being said in order to gain a broader understanding of the forces that have shaped the individual both in the past and presently.

KEEPING AN OPEN MIND

Assessments should be open, meaning that clinicians should not foreclose learning and openness by drawing conclusions prematurely—before they have a full picture of what is happening.

Part of being open means keeping blame out of the assessment (Bowlby, 1988). Clinicians should avoid blaming parents for problems they have experienced in their lives. A clinician who approaches a family with a stance of blame will be prone to look solely for risks rather than to see real and potential strengths that a parent may bring to the caregiving role. The clinician will have difficulties in appraising the situation in a differentiated manner and, as a result, may draw premature or biased conclusions about risk and competency. Importantly, a clinician who comes in with a negative stance may act in ways that criticize, devalue, threaten, or undermine families.

Therefore, personal biases and prejudices must be recognized and put aside in any assessment. This means approaching families without negative labels or blame attached to mental illness and without preconceptions about the relationship between mental illness and parenting capability, about whether children should be raised by biological versus foster parents, and about the outcome of the assessment. Although remaining open is essential, it does not mean being blind to actual risks or dangers.

Steps that can be taken to ensure that a clinician approaches an assessment with an open mind to learning include the following: being alert to one's own biases, including his or her theoretical principles and personal beliefs about parents, child maltreatment, mental illness, and assessments; listening to what families and others have to say; thoughtful questioning about what is not clear; and team discussions about one's own and other potential biases. Ongoing questioning coupled with an exploration and probing of one's own thoughts, hopes, and feelings about a particular assessment and its outcome are part of a process that can further openness (Gilkerson & Shahmoon-Shanok, 2000). In this endeavor, assessors should gather as much information as possible on a parent and family before making up their minds about a given situation (Lieberman, 1990).

A MULTIDISCIPLINARY APPROACH

Assessing the parenting capabilities of individuals with major mental illness calls for a multidisciplinary and integrative team approach. Individuals who assess parenting competency come from various disciplines—social work, psychiatry (adult or child), psychology (clinical and developmental), pediatrics, psychiatric nursing, counseling, sociology, criminal justice, and law. Some may be home visitors who work to support at-risk families. In conducting an assessment, clinicians draw on the areas of knowledge outlined in Table 3.1. Findings from these diverse areas are integrated, or put together, during the assessment.

One advantage of a multidisciplinary team is that members can scrutinize information from different viewpoints, providing both a more comprehensive view and a multilayered, in-depth approach. Team members who come from different disciplines can further understanding by placing findings in a fresh perspective or by pointing out relevant but overlooked issues that need to be addressed. A multidisciplinary team is also in an ideal position to probe interpretations, integrate findings, understand larger systemic influences on parenting and children, and make integrative recommendations that can benefit the parents' and children's health and well-being.

Forming a multidisciplinary team may not always be feasible. In rural areas, for instance, agencies may be lucky to have one social worker or medical doctor who is responsible for addressing the pressing mental health issues in

Table 3.1. Foundation knowledge for parenting assessments

Diagnosis and treatment of psychiatric disorders
Maternal mental illness in relation to parenting and child development
Assessment of parenting (various domains)
Child and adolescent assessment
Assessment of parent-child attachment bond
Assessment of social network
Dynamics of family violence and child maltreatment
Knowledge of the state child protective system
Forensics
State laws regarding parental and child rights

the region. In other instances, workloads may not allow for the formation of specialized, multidisciplinary teams. In cases in which a multidisciplinary team is not feasible, a mental health professional can broaden understanding by consulting with others who have expertise in specific areas.

In one situation, a pediatrician from a rural region was able to address multidisciplinary issues: The pediatrician was treating a young infant born to a mother with schizoaffective disorder, a disorder in which an individual shows some symptoms of schizophrenia but also experiences major depressive episodes and/or mania. When issues arose about the mother's difficulty in engaging the baby in face-to-face play, the pediatrician corresponded with a clinical child psychologist on a regular basis so as to better understand how the mother's mental illness might be having an impact on her ability to care for her newborn. Of particular interest was determining how at risk the baby was due to the mother's lack of engagement. A social worker was later engaged to monitor both the mother and the baby in the home. As part of the consultation, the team discussed the availability of other supports (e.g., relatives, neighbors, church members) and the viability of home visits and monitoring by a nearby agency. A psychiatrist from a nearby clinic provided consultation on the mother's medication. Consultation between this more informal multidisciplinary team continued for about 1 year and led to the infant remaining safely in the mother's care.

ARTICULATING QUESTIONS THAT MATTER

Assessments are only as useful as the questions that are formulated. Useful assessments, then, address questions that matter. They are tailored to address the specific needs raised by an individual family and articulate questions that bring families, service coordinators, and others involved with the family further with regard to understanding, decision making, and planning.

A good way to articulate questions that matter is to create an open dialogue at the outset that clarifies why an assessment is needed at this particular point in time. The initial steps of this process are illustrated in the next vignette, which involves a conversation between a caseworker and clinician. Ms. Albertson, who is the client, lost custody of her children following an episode of major depression. During that time, her children missed school for several weeks.

Clinician: What are your main concerns about Ms. Albertson?

Service coordinator: If you ask me, she still seems to be depressed. She cries a lot and doesn't like to go outside. She has also missed a few visits with the kids, even though I know that they are important to her. On other occasions, though, I wonder if she really is depressed. At times, she seems overly cheerful, even giddy.

Clinician: You seem to be telling me that sometimes Ms. Albertson doesn't seem depressed. Tell me more about why you are thinking this.

Service coordinator: Well, Ms. Albertson's moods change from one day to the next. She is depressed one day, and then the next day she is talkative and cheerful. She talks so fast that I can hardly follow her. I also worry about her finances because she spends a lot of money at times. She is so upbeat that she doesn't sleep much either. Last week, for instance, she took the children on a long drive at midnight.

Clinician: Has she been seen by a psychiatrist recently?

Service coordinator: Well, she did have a psychiatric evaluation when her children were taken away, but that was more than 8 months ago. At that time, major depression was diagnosed.

In this scenario, it becomes clear early on that Ms. Albertson is experiencing new psychiatric symptoms that are having an impact on her parenting. Getting a psychiatric evaluation could help to clarify her actual diagnosis. If she has bipolar disorder rather than clinical depression, she might not be getting the right medications.

The following types of questions may help clinicians to check whether the questions they are formulating are meaningful and answerable (Herbert & Harper-Dorton, 2002): What is unclear in this referral? Why have these problems arisen, and why do they persist? What is to be addressed and answered? Will an assessment answer this question and help the family and others to better understand the effects of mental illness on parenting? Can I answer these questions, or is another type of assessment better able to address them?

CLARIFYING ROLES

At the outset of an assessment, a clinician should clarify the purpose of the assessment and spell out what his or her role is to all participants. Defining roles and expectations creates helpful boundaries so the client and others know what to expect. Boundary crossings and boundary violations should be avoided. Boundary crossings and violations usually involve countertransference enactments that may initially seem benign (Gabbard, 2000).

Some indications of boundary violations occur if the clinician feels excessively sorry for a client and spends more time than usual with that person, if he or she promises that the results of the assessment will be favorable to the client, or if the clinician begins to disclose his or her own problems to a client.

The more alive a clinician is to issues of countertransference and boundary problems, the better he or she will be able to avoid the pitfalls (Bowlby, 1988). To establish and define relationships and roles, assessors should do the following:

1. Explain the purpose and scope of the assessment in a way that is clear and understandable to all participants.

2. Explain to family members the limits of confidentiality. This means telling participants that relevant information they share during the assessment will be included in a report, if this is the case, as well as letting family members know that any information they share about risk, either to themselves or others, may require action on the part of the assessor because he or she is a mandated reporter.

3. Tell families what types of records and information will be gathered, who will gather this information, and why this information is needed.

4. Get written permission to obtain relevant information from records and from collateral historians.

5. Let participants know when they will hear about the results and to whom the findings will go.

6. Emphasize that they are open to answering or clarifying any questions families may have about the assessment process, findings, or recommendations.

MINIMIZING BIAS

A particular challenge for assessors is to ensure that the information they gather is objective. Bias can enter into an assessment in various ways. A common source of bias results when information is gathered at an isolated point in time or if it is based only on the perspective of one person. For instance, a therapist who sees a mother with her child at the time when the mother is acutely depressed is likely to view her parenting skills quite differently than a therapist who has worked closely with the mother for several months and has seen the strides she has taken in understanding her own needs as well as her children's. Information about the mother's parenting from each perspective and at each point in time may reveal an important aspect of the larger picture. However, it is also limited because it is based only on partial information.

Another source of bias occurs if an assessor focuses his or her efforts on identifying risks that a parent poses to children without considering the competencies and strengths that the individual brings to the parenting role (Ackerson, 2003; Budd & Holdsworth, 1996). Although it is critical to determine risks, most parents will show flaws or weaknesses in their parenting when under close scrutiny. Almost all parents have strengths as well, and these need to be factored in to gain a holistic view of parenting competency and risk.

When an assessment is undertaken to address issues about child custody, bias can enter in due to the adversarial context in which such assessments occur. A mother in this situation may try to portray herself in the best light possible so as to keep her children. If parents are separated, divorced, or at odds with each other, a parent may try to portray the other parent's mental health and caregiving skills in negative ways so as to strengthen his or her own position.

Assessments cannot completely eliminate bias. The following steps, however, can be taken to help clinicians minimize bias:

1. Conduct independent assessments rather than assessments that support a specific viewpoint.

2. Employ multiple data collection methods, and draw on multiple sources of data so as to contribute to credible findings and interpretations through triangulation.

3. Be aware of your own biases, and discuss possible biases in team meetings.

4. Challenge yourself to look at findings from different perspectives.

5. Assess families in different contexts and allow adequate time to learn about parenting in different contexts.

6. Make sure that weaknesses are viewed in relation to a parent's strengths.

7. Write extensive notes on each session or record sessions so as to have documentation on different parts of the assessment.

8. Examine all available data with an open mind before drawing conclusions about risk and competency.

USING TOOLS THAT PROVIDE VALID AND USEFUL INFORMATION

Utilizing measures that provide valid and useful information is another essential part of an assessment. Assessors should also do the following things:

1. Establish which standard of parenting (excellent, good enough, minimal) needs to be assessed, and select tools that are geared to distinguish this standard.

2. Select measures that can be used to inform planning and decision-making for this particular individual or family (Shonkoff, 2000).

3. Rely on multiple tools and multiple sources of data.

4. Choose measures that can provide valid and reliable information for the family being seen.

5. Select measures that can be completed in a reasonable amount of time and that are not too long or demanding in the context of a lengthy assessment.

6. Determine whether the measures are relevant for evaluating the stage of parenting or development under assessment.

Before assessors decide to use one measure or the other, they should consider the context of use, the information source (e.g., mother, her partner, child), the theoretical framework of the measure, how easily the measure can be interpreted (how specialized or complicated it is), its standardization, and what the issues are of training and cost.

ASSESSING PARENTING DIRECTLY

The best way to evaluate parenting behavior is to observe a parent and child in naturally occurring, everyday situations (Hynan, 2003; Meisels, 2001). Unfortunately, many current assessments do not make observations the centerpiece of the assessment. Rather, they rely on projective measures or other tests that measure individual psychological or psychiatric functioning and that are only indirectly relevant, if at all, to parenting capacity (Budd & Holdsworth, 1996). A parent with a mental illness may demonstrate responses that can be interpreted as psychopathology on such a measure, yet still be a capable parent.

One reason for the frequent use of indirect measures may stem from the belief that alleged perpetrators of child maltreatment cannot be counted on to openly acknowledge or show their own risk behaviors. Some parents, however, do not hide such behaviors. Moreover, direct observations of parent–child interactions can be difficult to fake because they rely on both the parents' and the children's behavior, which has developed in response to repeated types of interactions with a parent.

Observation of a parent interacting with his or her child provides the most direct information on a parent's caregiving skills: how a mother protects her child from harm, whether she can prioritize her child's needs over her own needs, whether she can provide the child with adequate food and clothing, and how she comforts her child and responds to stress. It also yields rich information on the quality and nature of the child's relationship to the parent and can tell an assessor how the child feels about the parent and whether he or she can express and share his or her feelings and thoughts openly with the parent.

Direct observations of parents and children should be interpreted using theory and research principles (Hynan, 2003). Moreover, assessors should be trained to focus on which dimensions are most important, what the optimal level of stress is, and how many sessions are needed.

CONTEXTUAL CONSIDERATIONS

In an assessment, care should be taken to observe the parent in different settings and over time to adjust for situational and contextual influences. A mother who is highly anxious and under scrutiny is likely to act somewhat differently than she would if she felt secure. Similarly, a child will act differently if he or she is ill on the day when the assessment is conducted. Children who have been separated may act quite differently because their feelings may change. Some children in this situation may be highly prone to please a parent; others may be anxious, silent, angry, guarded, or unable to recognize the parent altogether (Bowlby, 1988). Asking the parent and others about whether an observation is typical and comparing observations with each other can help to ensure that the findings are valid.

Some contexts provide more valuable information than other situations on parenting behavior. Because stress is an important contributor to parenting breakdown and child maltreatment (Belsky, 1993), it is helpful to observe a mother in a stressful context with her children in an assessment. This, when coupled with naturalistic observations in other settings, can help the assessor understand a mother's ability to cope and to prioritize her children's needs.

MAKING ASSESSMENTS DEVELOPMENTALLY RELEVANT

The skills that a mother needs to care for a young infant differ from the skills that she will need to care for a toddler or an older child. The mother of a young infant will need to have the stamina to get up several times at night for feedings and be emotionally available to respond to the baby's communication and bids for attention. A mother of a toddler must be alert to her child's growing sense of independence and selfhood. She must be able to deal with the formidable temper tantrums that characterize this age group and meet her child's need for closeness and protection (Lieberman, 1993). Caring for a school-age child requires monitoring and support as the child engages with peers and establishes his or her developmental competencies in the real world (Sroufe, 1995). Caring for an adolescent will require attending to the adolescent's needs for autonomy, identity, and mixed-gender relationships. Caring for a large family of children or for a child with special developmental or medical needs will require other parenting skills.

It follows that assessments need to address what is required by a parent to care for children of different ages and with different needs (Sroufe, 1995). For infants and young children, critical areas to assess include the quality and nature of the child's attachment bond to his or her caregivers; his or her ability to use, explore, and negotiate the environment; and his or her emerging language and cognitive skills (see Table 3.2). Assessing the quality of the parent–child relationship remains an important part of the assessment of older children. However, other domains also move into the foreground. For school-age children, important developmental domains to assess include a child's relationship to school and academic achievement, his or her sense of self, and the quality of peer friendships. Issues of delinquency may be important concerns in adolescence (Tolan et al., 2003).

Some parenting skills are necessary components of parenting children at all age levels. A mother's ability to handle stress, to form and maintain

Table 3.2. Caregiving skills needed to address children's developmental needs

Age	Issue	Role for caregiver
0–3 months	Physiological regulation (turning toward)	Smooth routines
3–6 months	Management of tension	Sensitive, cooperative interaction
6–12 months	Establishing an effective attachment relationship	Responsive availability
12–18 months	Exploration and mastery	Secure base
18–30 months	Individuation (autonomy)	Firm support
30–54 months	Management of impulses, sex-role identification, peer relations	Clear roles, values; flexible self-control
6–11 years	Consolidating self-concept, loyal friendships, effective same-gender peer group functioning, real-world competence	Monitoring, supporting activities, co-regulation
Adolescence	Personal identify, mixed-gender relationships, intimacy	Available resource, monitor the child's ability to monitor himself

From Sroufe, L.A. (1995). *Emotional development: The organization of emotional life in the early years.* Cambridge, England: Cambridge University Press; adapted by permission.

supportive relationships with others, and to be sensitive to the needs and individualities of others are examples of more constant skills from which a parent will need to draw in caring for children of all ages. Assessing what is developmentally relevant, then, includes examining the more constant skills that comprise good enough parenting, assessing the unique skills that are needed to care for each individual child, and assessing a mother's ability to adapt to her child's changing needs over time.

ANCHORING CONCLUSIONS IN PATTERNS

A parenting assessment draws on information from multiple sources in order to assess the competencies and risks that a mother brings to the parenting role. It synthesizes this information in a critical way to elucidate how mental illness symptoms affect an individual's parenting skills both in the past and presently (Göpfert, Webster, & Seeman, 2004). Critical contexts and factors that may impede or facilitate parenting are also articulated so as to obtain a holistic picture of parenting competency and risk.

To achieve these aims, conclusions that are drawn about parenting need to be based on patterns of behavior, thoughts, and feelings that are observed across different time periods and in different contexts. Assessors can begin the process of identifying larger patterns, or themes, about parenting and mental illness by scrutinizing all available data for consistencies and inconsistencies. Identifying consistent patterns in an assessment provides the foundation for determining the risks and strengths that a mother brings to the parenting task. Identifying inconsistencies, by contrast, points to areas in which more information and clarification will be needed to complete the assessment.

APPROACHING INTERPRETATIONS CAUTIOUSLY

If an assessment is done well, it is based on observations and draws on a variety of methods and measures. It looks at parenting in different contexts. An array of factors—psychiatric, environmental, treatment—that can influence parenting are also considered.

This approach allows assessors to describe past and present parenting behaviors, draw conclusions about larger patterns, and understand contexts that influence parenting for better or worse. Assessors can also comment on parenting risks and strengths, interventions that may help, the barriers to change, and the likelihood of change occurring in the near future (Budd & Holdsworth,1996).

Even with a best-practices approach to assessment, assessors should be aware that they do not have all of the information or knowledge about risk and competency. Predicting future behavior is always difficult as predictions involve probability estimates that can change over time. Predicting too far into the future is impossible. Therefore, it is essential for assessors to give an honest brokering of knowledge and uncertainties (Gambrill, 2006) and to approach interpretations about future parenting competency and risk with caution.

KEEPING CONSEQUENCES IN MIND

Assessments provide critical data for decision making and planning (Budd et al., 2001). A judge may conclude from an assessment that a mother is not able to care for her children and that she is unlikely to change her parenting skills in a time frame that makes sense for her child. As a result of this conclusion, the judge may sign papers that will terminate parental rights. In this case, the child may grow up as a ward of the state or be placed in long-term foster care.

Given the far-reaching consequences of assessments, assessors should do the following:

1. Obtain the prerequisite knowledge, training, and expertise to interpret findings and instruments and to evaluate parenting competency.

2. Address only the questions that they can competently answer.

3. Make sure findings are based on patterns that are observed over time and in different contexts.

4. Write clear, balanced reports that explain findings and diagnoses in lay terms.

5. Do not overstate findings or conclusions.

6. Understand the limitations of prediction and underscore such limitations in reports.

7. Ensure that reports give due consideration to a parent's potential for change.

8. Complete assessments, reports, and feedback sessions in a timely manner so as to facilitate understanding, decision-making, and planning.

COUPLING ASSESSMENTS WITH INTERVENTIONS

Even the most comprehensive assessment will not be useful unless it is followed up with recommendations that are meaningful—recommendations that address a family's specific situation and needs (Herbert & Harper-Dorton, 2003; Meisels, 2001). The process of linking conclusions of an assessment to recommendations starts with outlining the areas of risk to target in an intervention. Based on this outline, the clinician then identifies specific interventions or therapy modalities that can help remediate each area of risk or weakness that is identified.

Interventions should be realistic and based on the knowledge of how a parent, individual, or family has responded to past interventions and how they are currently responding to treatment (if applicable). Interventions that are recommended should also be available in the community in which the individuals reside. In addition, they should be based on scientific evidence and reflect the most up-to-date knowledge about the effectiveness of the intervention and service (Briggs & Rzepnicki, 2004; Corcoran, 2000). Considering parents' strengths and their points of view about what is important to them should guide the feedback process at all points.

Some assessments spell out which interventions should be prioritized and which are the most critical to start with so as to help families onto healthier pathways. Prioritizing interventions is important when families have multiple needs or if one intervention has logical precedence over others.

4

The Assessment Process

An assessment of parenting competency and risk includes direct observations of parent–child interactions; a psychiatric evaluation; consideration of the parent's home environment and social support network; an assessment of children's developmental, emotional, and attachment needs; and a record review. Examining how a parent has responded to past interventions and under what conditions parenting could change is part of the assessment. In the assessment process, patterns and discrepancies in the data are identified through the process of triangulation—information from one source is confirmed from information with other sources. Conclusions about competency and risk are then drawn, and recommendations are made for interventions to help parents and children onto healthier pathways. Underlying the assessment process is a conceptual and empirical understanding of how mental illness symptoms can affect parenting and child development and how different contexts and situations can evoke parenting risk behavior.

This chapter outlines the process of assessment. Drawing on attachment, ecological, and violence risk potential theories, the chapter contains a conceptual framework for understanding the dynamics of parenting competency and risk. Next, various aspects of the assessment process are described: parenting domains to assess, the team composition, intake procedures, how assessors come to conclusions, and report writing. The chapter then includes a discussion on countertransference issues, court testimony, and crisis situations.

UNDERSTANDING PARENTING COMPETENCY AND RISK

Attachment theory, ecological theory, and violence risk prediction theory provide a rich conceptual framework for understanding parenting competency and risk in individuals with mental illness. Attachment theory provides a basis for understanding the bonds of love that bind the parent and child to each other and why a parent takes care of a child in the particular way he or she does. It emphasizes the parent's own attachment history and the role of the parent's current state of mind toward these experiences as major determinants of parenting (Bowlby, 1988; Solomon & George, 1996).

Ecological theory underscores that parenting breakdown and parenting risk are multiply determined (Belsky, 1984, 1993; Cicchetti & Toth, 1995). According to this theory, an assessment of parenting competency looks at a comprehensive array of theory-based risk factors in multiple domains of functioning. Focus is given to the role of parental and child characteristics, intergenerational and family dynamics, the home environment, and cultural and societal factors in compromising or promoting a parent's ability to nurture and provide adequate care and protection to children.

Violence risk potential theory (Monahan, 1996; Steadman & Monahan, 2001) looks at the component parts of risk (i.e., variables that predict violence). It underscores the need to assess a rich array of theoretically relevant risk factors with attention given to factors that have been specifically linked to violence or harm (Monahan, 1996). The factors that this theory focus on include a mother's childhood experiences, her current disposition (e.g., angry, impulsive, psychopathic), and situations that could evoke risk behaviors. Careful examination is given to the contribution of specific mental illness symptoms—delusions, hallucinations, or violent fantasies—to violence risk potential, as well as the course and prognosis of the illness and the individual's responsiveness and compliance with treatment. In this theory, risk is viewed as a probability estimate that can change over time and in different contexts.

Figure 4.1 depicts an integrative model of parenting competency and risk. In this figure, parenting competency and parenting breakdown are viewed as different end results of the complex interplay between parenting skills, mental illness factors, and environmental, child, and attachment factors that interact with each other in complex ways to reduce or potentiate risk. For example, a mother who has had rejecting and abusive experiences in

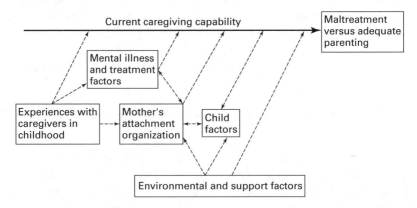

Figure 4.1. Determinants of caregiving capability in mothers with mental disorders. (From Jacobsen, T. [2004]. Mentally ill mothers in the parenting role: Clinical management and treatment. In M. Göpfert, J. Webster, & M.V. Seeman [Eds.], *Parental psychiatric disorder: Distressed parents and their families* [2nd ed.; p. 113]. England: Cambridge University Press; reprinted by permission.)

childhood and who remains traumatized by those experiences is more likely to be vulnerable to the stresses of parenting should she meet with seriously adverse events. Her risk would be further increased if she was depressed and refused treatment or had a child with special needs. Risk would be decreased if the mother was engaged in therapy, had good insight into her illness, had good coping skills, and had a viable network of people who could help her in the parenting role.

CONTENT AREAS TO ASSESS

The model depicted in Figure 4.1 provides a template for the assessment, which focuses first and foremost on the quality and nature of a mother's caregiving skills. Parenting encompasses a broad range of abilities. It includes a mother's ability to meet her child's needs for physical care and protection, nurturance, and love; how and the extent to which she helps set limits; how she helps her child to master and organize experiences, and her ability to recognize when her child's needs are met (Magura & Moses, 1986).

To assess parenting capability and risk, clinicians observe the nature and quality of parent–child interactions in different settings, review records to obtain information on a mother's parenting in the past, and find out how a mother feels about her child and her parenting. Inquiry is also made into how a mother understands her child's individual needs, how she empathizes with her child, and how well she understands child-rearing practices, including her disciplinary practices.

As illustrated in Figure 4.1, assessors also obtain information on contextual influences (i.e., factors internal and external to the mother that have an impact on parenting quality). Because parenting is strongly influenced by a mother's experiences with her own attachment figures in childhood, one contextual area to explore involves the experiences that a mother had with her caregivers over the years of infancy, childhood, and adolescence. Particular inquiry is made into experiences of support and comfort and also into experiences of loss, abandonment, and maltreatment (Bowlby, 1988; Egeland, Bosquet, & Chung, 2002). The mother's state of mind about attachment experiences is also relevant to a parenting assessment as it tells an assessor how a mother currently processes and thinks about attachment relationships. For instance, if a mother continues to be traumatized by past experiences or remains highly insecure about the availability of others, then her own attachment needs may take priority over parenting (Bowlby, 1988). This process is illustrated in the next vignette.

In childhood, Lorna experienced long periods of time during which she was left alone. Her mother was seriously depressed and was so absorbed in her own pain that she often did not note Lorna's needs. As a result, when Lorna became upset or distraught in adulthood, she needed a great deal of support from others to calm down. It was only when other individuals were available to meet her needs that Lorna was able to note her children's distress and needs.

As part of the assessment, clinicians examine a mother's ability to respond to stress, her emotional maturity and stability (Egeland, Carlson, & Sroufe, 1993), and her coping skills and other aspects of her personality, including her intellectual functioning. Mothers who fare well in the parenting role are socially adept, show good ability to plan, and can invest themselves emotionally in other people and maintain healthy relationships (Bowlby, 1988).

The mother's psychiatric illness is another important context to assess. Illness dimensions and symptoms are usually more important predictors of parenting risk than psychiatric diagnoses (Goodman & Emory, 1992; Sameroff, Seifer, & Zax, 1982). Indeed, several mental illness symptoms have been found to increase the risk of parenting breakdown. Active psychotic symptoms in a mother; delusions that include a child; rapidly changing mental states; the presence of aggressive, violent, or suicidal behavior; deteriorating judgment; and a concomitant substance addiction can all increase the risk that a mother will neglect or abuse a child (Jacobsen & Miller, 1998b; Kumar et al., 1995). Illness severity and chronicity as well as a concomitant addiction are other mental illness factors that can negatively influence parenting outcome (Alpern & Lyons-Ruth, 1993), whereas good insight into her illness can ameliorate risk (Mullick, Miller, & Jacobsen, 2001). Each of these areas is given consideration in the psychiatric evaluation.

Parenting is a stressful job that is best accomplished with support from others. If family members and friends are available to step in to aid a mother in times of stress and to provide her with needed emotional support, she is far more likely to be able to muster the necessary resources and energy to devote to parenting than a mother who lacks support (Coohey, 1996).

Family members can have adverse effects on parenting as well, especially if relationships are dysfunctional or violent (Kitzmann, Gaylord, Holt, & Kenny, 2003; Tajima, 2000). Adverse effects are more common if the parent has ongoing contact with abusive family members (Bowlby, 1988) and in cases in which relatives reinforce the sick role and fail to consult a mother in making decisions about children (Nicholson et al., 1998a). Therefore, assessing support networks is an essential part of a parenting assessment. Other environmental factors to assess include the family's economic status, sudden changes in family life and family organization, ongoing crises, family moves, poor health, and disability (Egeland et al., 1993).

Table 4.1. Content areas to cover in parenting assessment

Parenting abilities
  Feelings, thoughts, and beliefs about parenting
  Ability to interact in a healthy and appropriate manner with her child
  Understanding of her children's individual needs and personality
  Ability to allow her child to grow (e.g., to master and organize the world)
  Emotional maturity and stability
  Ability to respond to and cope with stress
  Current state of mind about attachment
  Childhood attachment experiences
Psychiatric factors
  Psychiatric symptoms (e.g., delusions, hallucinations, anger, impulsiveness)
  Suicidal or homicidal thoughts or actions
  Insight into illness
  Presence of a concomitant addiction
  Course and prognosis of the illness
  Treatment responsiveness and compliance
Environmental stressors and support
  Number of children the mother is raising
  Presence of domestic or family violence
  Social support
  Economic resources
  Whether the mother is an adolescent or mother for the first time
The child's needs
  Attachment quality to parent and other significant individuals
  Emotional, social, and cognitive functioning
  Major medical or psychiatric problems; learning or developmental delays

Assessors also look at children's needs as they provide information on how a child has fared in the parent's care. If a child has been seriously neglected by a parent, the neglect will have an impact on his or her cognitive and linguistic skills as well as how the child relates to others. Children are never responsible for maltreatment. Nonetheless, special needs or behavior problems in a child need to be considered as they can increase parental stress and raise the level of parenting risk (Belsky, 1993; Sullivan & Knutson, 2000). When the assessment is successfully completed, a clinician should have rich information on the various content areas described in Table 4.1.

WHICH DISCIPLINES TO INCLUDE?

To obtain a holistic view of the family and of risk and protective factors that contribute to parenting quality, a multidisciplinary and integrative approach is essential. Clinicians with expertise in psychiatry, parenting, child development, pediatrics, and social work conduct assessments. The exact constitution of a team may vary, however, depending on the questions raised by the family being seen. In general, the choice of the team composition (both size and area of expertise) is guided by three sets of parameters: the questions to be addressed, who has the expertise to address the questions, and the complexity and scope of the case.

If the mother has a young baby, the team might include a pediatrician and psychiatric social worker. If the mother has already had a recent comprehensive psychiatric evaluation, the team could include a psychologist with expertise in parenting along with a psychiatric social worker. In complicated cases, a professional team of members from three or four disciplines may be needed. For example, if a mother has several children with varying levels of medical and psychological needs, has lost custody of her children, or has major questions about the nature of her psychiatric symptoms and treatment, an interdisciplinary team that includes a pediatrician, a psychiatrist, and a social worker may be needed to interpret the data.

Teams will benefit from a coordinator who conducts the intake assessment, gathers relevant data, coordinates meetings, and writes the summary report. Any team member can do this job, but it should be clear that this position requires considerable time engagement.

CHARACTERISTICS OF TEAM MEMBERS

Beyond expertise in their specific disciplines, team members should possess the following characteristics (Miller et al., 1998):

- Good personal skills
- The ability to interact meaningfully with a variety of individuals, including those in crisis
- The ability to interact well with other team members
- The ability to work independently
- Excellent verbal, written, and communicative skills
- Sensitivity to cultural considerations
- Flexibility
- Self-reflection
- The ability to take a systemic perspective
- The ability and willingness to learn from different perspectives
- Good organizational skills
- Sound assessment skills
- Good knowledge of community resources

INTAKE PROCEDURES

An intake with a family service coordinator or other professional initiates the assessment process. Typically, a referral is made from another mental health professional or child welfare service coordinator, although family members, a judge, or an attorney could also initiate an assessment. The intake process determines which specific questions are to be addressed, whether the team has the expertise to assess these questions, and whether the referral falls in the purview of the team's expertise.

Questions that are formulated should be specific and answerable. The following are relevant questions for a parenting assessment team:

- What is Ms. K's current *DSM-IV-TR* diagnosis?

- How does Mrs. L's history and present behavior affect her ability to parent?

- Does Ms. C demonstrate adequate parenting skills to safely care for her children?

- How do Mrs. S's psychiatric symptoms affect her parenting capabilities?

- Which objective tasks does Ms. B need to complete before her child could be returned home?

- What is the optimal treatment for Ms. M to maintain psychiatric stability?

- Is Mrs. P aware of her need for treatment, including the need for continued treatment if she regains custody of her children?

- How do Mrs. R's children fare emotionally when she is clinically depressed?

If the questions do not lie in the competency of the team or if the case is not appropriate, the team coordinator identifies resources for the referred individual (e.g., an agency or individual who is able to address the questions at hand).

Gathering all pertinent records (e.g., psychiatric, child, school, child welfare) is a central part of the intake process. Records provide an important and essential perspective to the assessment, telling assessors about a parent's functioning or parenting at other periods of time. Data from these sources will be compared to information gathered in interviews and observations. Triangulation, or the process of comparing information from one source with information from other sources, is a critical part of the assessment process because it contributes to a more holistic, balanced, and comprehensive perspective of competency and risk.

Once a case is accepted, the next step is to clarify the nature of the assessment to participants, obtain their informed consent to participate, and give the referred individual and family a time when the assessment will be conducted and completed (Miller et al., 1998). Informed consent is based on the particular individual's understanding of what the assessment will entail and to what they are giving permission. It includes understanding that there is no promise as to the outcome and that the participant can stop the assessment and drop out at any time unless the assessment is mandated by a judge. In cases involving the court, letting the parent and child know that the team does not decide on custody but provides information to the judge to make informed decisions is essential. Letting the parent and other family members know that the assessor and team are neutral, and ensuring that this is the case, are other important parts of the process.

To obtain records, the coordinator contacts the relevant agency and finds out the process for sending records. Obtaining records requires getting consent forms from the parent. Keeping a tracking system for consents and records facilitates a timely completion of the assessment. The following records are likely to be relevant to an assessment:

- Psychiatric records
- Psychological evaluations
- Psychosocial histories
- Developmental and psychological assessments of children
- Children's school records and tests
- Child welfare records
- Criminal background checks

If a mother has had numerous psychiatric hospitalizations, obtaining accurate information on the names of the hospitals, their locations, and the treating professionals is likely to be difficult. Compiling a list of all of the hospitals in the area may be one way to help a mother recall the places she has been. Often, information on past hospitalizations can be gathered if the team tracks recent hospital records and checks whether such records list prior hospitals where a mother was admitted (Miller et al., 1998).

Separate consents are needed to contact collateral historians and for criminal background checks. Special consent is also needed if the assessor plans to videotape a session or to obtain an audio recording of interviews.

LENGTH OF EVALUATIONS

Assessments typically occur over four to six sessions. The length of the parenting assessment will vary, however, depending on the size of the family and

Table 4.2.   Estimated time needed to complete
assessments

Assessment	Estimated time
Psychiatric	
Interview	1–2 hours
Interview with collateral historians	1–2 hours
Record review	1–2 hours
Report writing	3 hours
Caregiving	
Interview and questionnaires	1–2 hours
Interview with collateral historians	1 hour
Record review	1–2 hours
Report writing	3 hours
Child	
Interview and observations	2–3 hours
Interview with collateral historians	1 hour
Record review	1–2 hours
Report writing	3 hours
Social history	
Home visit and interview	2–3 hours
Interview with collateral historians	1 hour
Record review	1–2 hours
Report writing	3 hours
Summary	
Report review	1–2 hours
Report writing	3 hours

the complexity of the issues to be addressed. If numerous questions need to be addressed, several children need to be assessed, and a large number of records need to be reviewed, the length of time to complete the assessment will be different than it will be for a mother with one child and fewer records. Table 4.2 provides an estimation of the time it will likely take assessors to complete the assessments.

TEAM MEETINGS

In regularly scheduled meetings, team members present findings on the psychiatric, caregiving, child, and social assessments. The meeting begins with the team coordinator presenting a brief synopsis of the purpose of the assessment and of the family's composition and background history. Following this, individual team members summarize their findings in a concise manner.

Once all of the findings have been presented, the team raises questions and discusses issues that are unclear and identifies patterns in the data. Inconsistencies usually indicate that more information is needed to understand the issues at hand. Once inconsistencies have been clarified, the next step involves formulating the main risk and protective factors that emerge from the data. This requires a consensus among team members who question and actively come to terms with all findings until the data are understood in a balanced and integrative manner. When the team reaches a consensus, recommendations are then discussed and hierarchized in the order of importance. During this phase, report writing begins. If a consensus is not achieved, then more data must be gathered to address questions that remain unclear.

Creating an atmosphere in which findings can be discussed openly is an essential ingredient of the team process (Miller et al., 1998). A lively, thoughtful, and open exchange characterizes well-functioning teams. Team members should listen to other viewpoints, play the devil's advocate, and integrate findings to build a more holistic and balanced perspective. In a team that works well, members discuss how their own views may affect their thinking and are aware of the powerful effects that some families may have on their feelings. Members of a well-functioning team are comfortable with sharing their feelings and thoughts with each other so as to better understand the situation at hand. If the team is too hierarchical, important findings may not be brought up in the first place or may be overlooked. Mutual respect, support, and the ability to openly disagree are other components that characterize a well-functioning team. Although hierarchies are to be discouraged, a coordinator who leads the team plays a key role in ensuring that discussions are open and balanced and that all perspectives are heard and represented.

Ideally, team members read each other's reports and provide feedback to ensure integration and to check for any factual or other errors. Reading each other's reports also helps to ensure that a summary report provides a factual, neutral, and comprehensive overview of the team's findings.

COMING TO CONCLUSIONS

In coming to conclusions, team members prioritize and weigh risk and protective factors (Steadman & Monahan, 2001). In the process of coming to conclusions, team members should view risk not as something static but as something that can change over time and in different contexts (Monahan, 1996). They should also consider the likelihood that the risk equation may change if optimal treatment is offered to the parent or child. Moreover, team members should recognize that risk factors can vary in their importance depending on their interactions with other risk factors.

Team members also consider the child's needs and best interest (Goldstein, Solnit, Goldstein, & Freud, 1998). The decision-making process examines what the child's pathway will be if the parent (and child) are engaged in therapy, and it examines the potential developmental pathways a child could take if he or she lives with or returns home to the parent (Bowlby, 1973). For example, if an intervention is likely to take 2 years to complete and the mother has a baby in foster care, the intervention may not match the child's interests because he or she will likely have established a primary attachment to the foster parent. A 2-year intervention for an adolescent living with an older sibling may have a smaller impact on the adolescent's well-being.

In looking at the child's needs, the assessor focuses on the fit between the child and parent. Can the parent meet this specific child's needs so that the child's psychological and physical well-being are taken into account? Can this parent assure that the child will be part of a family in which "she feels wanted and will have the opportunity, on a continuing basis, to receive and return affection, as well as to express anger and learn to manage aggression" (Goldstein et al., 1998, p. 6)?

Based on the findings, team members may then decide by consensus whether to assign a higher- or lower-risk category (Mullick et al., 2001). The procedure used in coming to consensus is comparable to the best-estimate technique (Fink, Bernstein, Handelsman, Foote, & Lovejoy, 1995). This technique involves clinicians working together to come up with the best estimate of psychiatric diagnoses.

Ratings of risk are usually done on a continuum that assesses both risk and the likelihood of a parent responding to interventions (Mullick et al., 2001). A higher rating indicates that even if the mother is offered and responds to interventions, the prognosis for adequate parenting capability in a reasonable time frame is poor. A mid-level rating means that the prognosis for parenting carries some risks but that risks could be substantially affected if the mother engages in and responds to interventions. A lower rating could mean that the level of risk posed to children is low and no interventions are needed. But it could also mean that if specific interventions are offered and accepted, there is a reasonable likelihood that a mother can meet her children's needs adequately and can become an effective caregiver. In making ratings, assessors should spell out what the risks are—both generally and for each individual child—how serious the risks are, and what conditions could increase or ameliorate the risks.

The conclusion of a report spells out the level of risk, but it also lists the risk and protective factors that were identified in the assessment. Factors are listed in order of their importance. Care is also taken to specify contexts and situations that potentiate or ameliorate risk (Cicchetti, Rogosch, & Toth, 1998). For instance, a mother may show good enough parenting, but only when she has a solid support network and is on psychotropic medication.

RECOMMENDATIONS

Once the risk level has been ascertained, team members formulate realistic interventions that can make a difference for individuals and families. This includes specifying the following items:

- Which interventions are likely to improve parent and child outcomes

- How the interventions are related to specific risk factors

- Whether the resources are available in the parent's community

- How long the interventions will take before observable changes occur

- Whether the changes can take place in a time frame that makes sense for each child in the family

Recommendations are about treatment opportunities, not about making decisions regarding custody or visitation. Judges make such decisions based on the information provided by the team and on other available information.

REPORT WRITING

Findings from assessments are communicated verbally to parents, but they are based on an integrative report that summarizes, in writing, the purpose of the assessment, its findings, and recommendations for treatment. Depending on the scope of the assessment, one summary report may be written or several reports may be written by assessors from different disciplines (e.g., psychiatric, social work, psychological). If separate reports are written, an interactive summary report should tie together the findings and address the specific referral questions. Recommendations should be included in the summary report rather than in the individual report. All reports should be numbered and kept together so that they are presented as a whole and not piecemeal (Miller et al., 1998).

In writing reports, clinicians should remember that the audience they are writing for is usually not made up of clinicians, but rather parents, service coordinators, attorneys, or other individuals involved with the family. Individuals who read the report may not understand technical terms (Budd & Holdsworth, 1996; Budd, Poindexter, Felix, & Naik-Polan, 2001).

Good reports describe contexts and focus on behavior. They reveal patterns, evaluate the reliability and validity of the information that is presented, discuss the limitations of the methodology and conclusions, and offer alternative explanations. In addition, they cautiously make predictions regarding the future when the predictions cannot be substantiated, but they are definitive when the findings are clear (Budd et al., 2001).

The following principles should also guide the writing process (Budd et al., 2001; Miller et al., 1998):

- At the top of the report, bold lettering should be used to explain that the report is confidential.

- The purpose of the report and questions should be explicitly stated. These questions usually come from the referral source.

- All data sources should be explicitly listed in the report. Data sources should include the assessor's name, his or her qualifications (degree[s]), and the date the assessment was completed.

- If reports are written by the multidisciplinary team, each individual report should list the reports of other team members so as to underscore the integrative nature of the assessment.

- Information from different sources should be marked in the reports so that the assessment is clear about the source of the information.

- Jargon should be avoided and care should be taken to explain all terminology, including all diagnoses or technical terms.

- The report focuses on facts and findings. Opinions should be marked as opinions.

Clinicians should remember that parents will read the report. Care should thus be given to writing the report in an objective and thoughtful way. Although it is important to state risks, they should be written in a neutral, nonjudgmental tone.

A summary report synthesizes information from the main assessment areas—psychiatric, caregiving, child, home environment, and support—so that it can stand on its own. Service coordinators and court personnel have little time, and they may only read the assessment summary. Making this report complete, concise, and consistent is key.

The summary report provides an overview of the team's findings, including the purpose of the evaluation, a summary of the findings, the parent's *DSM-IV-TR* diagnosis, a summary of the children's needs, a summary of factors that lower the risk for neglect, an evaluation of the mother's caregiving capabilities, recommended interventions for each family member, and a time frame for a follow-up. The summary report should be written in a concise manner. It should be balanced, referencing both risks and strengths. The following hints may help in preparing this report (Budd et al., 2001):

- Determine what to put in this report after reviewing individual reports and identifying consistent patterns in the data set.

- Highlight the major areas of discussion in a logical order.

- Limit the report to four or five pages.

- Talk with other team members about any questions or differences they may have before finalizing this report.

- Remember that this report could serve as a legal document.

COMMUNICATING FINDINGS TO FAMILIES

Parents are given oral and written feedback on the findings from the assessment. The feedback session should allow enough time for the parent to not only hear the findings but also ask questions and receive clarification. Between 1 ½ and 2 hours is usually an adequate time frame to achieve these goals. The assessor should be prepared to provide the feedback in a neutral way and without apprehension, being as clear as possible about the findings and how they are linked to the overall conclusions and recommendations. The feedback session should cover risks and strengths (Miller et al., 1998).

In the session, assessors should avoid blame, even if a parent played a role in neglecting or harming a child. The assessment should be framed in terms of the family's needs and concerns, as this often opens doors for families to engage in interventions (Lieberman, Compton, Van Horn, & Ghosh Ippen, 2003).

The conclusion of the report and recommendations for treatment are central parts of the feedback to parents. Assessors should gauge beforehand how a parent will likely respond to feedback. If a mother is depressed and is likely to become suicidal, then steps should be put in place to ensure her safety. Like the assessment, the feedback session can provide an opportunity for early therapeutic intervention. Optimally, it will create a safe environment in which the parent receives clear feedback and recommendations for treatment strategies that will make a difference for the parent and family. Understanding the parent's perceptions and framing the intervention in terms of such perceptions is essential for ensuring the likelihood that the treatment will be taken seriously. Recommended treatment should be framed in the context of discussing the stresses and difficult circumstances that a family is going through (Lieberman et al., 2003).

WHEN TO FOLLOW UP

If specific recommendations are listed in the report as potentially changing the risk assessment, then a time frame should be stated as to when measurable changes might be expected to occur. At that time, a follow-up evaluation is scheduled to see whether the expected changes have occurred.

Recommendations about therapy should be specific. For example, the assessor should state what type of therapy is indicated for the area to address (e.g., cognitive or psychodynamic therapy). Although the goals of therapy should be specified, it is not wise to spell out in detail every issue to be covered or the length and time of each individual therapy session. These issues are best left for the therapist working with the parent, child, or family.

COURT TESTIMONY

Assessors may be required to testify in court, especially if a family has Child Protective Services involvement and if custody issues are at stake. Clinicians who have not testified in court should be aware of the adversarial stance they are likely to encounter once they are in the courtroom. One lawyer represents the parents' interests, another is there representing the child's interests. Each lawyer may try to selectively present data to highlight his or her position. An assessor should always remain neutral. This means evaluating the family without a promise about the outcome of the assessment and without receiving a fee for services as an expert witness. The team could be paid directly by the court or child welfare agency for services. If contacted by a lawyer to testify, the assessors should state at the outset that they will call it as they see it (Miller et al., 1998).

For the court testimony, the assessor should prepare in advance and be knowledgeable about all aspects of the reports, including dates. Assessors typically submit their vitae to the court and can expect to be questioned on dates when degrees were obtained and their expertise in the areas under question.

Because assessors testify without papers in hand, there is much to hold in mind before appearing in court. Once on the stand, an assessor should state that his or her "memory is exhausted" if he or she doesn't remember important details. An attorney will then ask what information might help to refresh his or her memory and at that time the assessor can request a copy of the report. Assessors should remember, however, that if notes are requested, these can be obtained by any lawyer who is working on the case, and such notes become part of the record of the case (Miller et al., 1998).

Prior to testifying in court, assessors should make sure they talk with lawyers who issue subpoenas to gain a sense of what the lawyer expects the assessors to address. Finding out what questions the lawyers will ask is wise. Assessors should view such meetings not as a way for lawyers to prepare them but as a way for the lawyers to help clarify what the assessor will talk about so the lawyers understand what information will be offered.

Being questioned or cross-examined in court can be intimidating. Clinicians should, therefore, keep in mind that they are experts. Time should be taken to formulate responses. Questions that require a "Yes" or "No" response are as common as pointed or misleading questions. Clinicians should listen carefully to each question. If questions are misleading, unclear, or skewed, clinicians should clarify what is being asked and should state what questions they can and cannot answer.

LEARNING FROM COUNTERTRANSFERENCE REACTIONS

Working with mothers who have mental illness and their families can take a toll on a clinician's well-being (Apfel & Handel, 1993). Issues of loss, guilt, parental rights, children's needs, illness and healing, relapse, and hospitalizations are recurrent themes that are revisited in different guises with each new assessment. Some clinicians are uncomfortable in the presence of mothers who are acutely psychotic (Apfel & Handel, 1993). Others may develop intense feelings if they treat a mother during pregnancy or in the postpartum period, worry about the baby's well-being, or feel that all children should stay with their parents. Yet for some clinicians, the themes of aggression, dependence, sexuality, and reproduction generate intense feelings that may be hard to cope with. Children who have become involved in a child protection agency can evoke strong feelings in clinicians as well, who may feel intense anger at what has happened (Jacobsen, Levy-Chung, & Kim, 2002). The unrealistic expectations of wishing to heal all, know all, and love all often underlie intense countertransference reactions (Eastwood, Spielvogel, & Wile, 1990).

Although assessors may have special difficulties as they wrestle with countertransference reactions, such feelings can provide valuable information about both the clinician and the issues facing the family. Therefore, examining these feelings in a supportive supervisory relationship is a critical part of the assessment process. Supervision that allows a clinician to reflect on his or her feelings about a family is a good place to begin the process of exploring intense countertransference reactions in a safe setting (Shahmoon-Shanok, Gilkerson, Eggbeer, & Fenichel, 1995).

The process of coming to terms with countertransference reactions involves an active search, discussion, and tolerance of feelings such as avoidance, anger, frustration, and envy. As clinicians can increase their respect for the powerful influence that parents with mental illness have on them, the more able they become to look beyond their preconceived notions of who these parents are and who they themselves are (Eastwood et al., 1990).

The team setting can offer another opportunity for clinicians who are enmeshed in countertransference patterns to explore troubling reactions and to hear clear, balanced perspectives from other team members (Eastwood et al., 1990). Time can be regularly set aside during team meetings to discuss and study various issues, such as grief, loss, parental rights, and children's needs, in greater depth. Articles about such issues may help a team to better understand the perspectives and views of others, thereby contributing to better understanding of the case (Eastwood et al., 1990).

CRISIS INTERVENTION

In some circumstances, clinicians find that the family they are assessing is in crisis and they will need to take swift action to avert risk. An assessment, for instance, may reveal that a mother requires immediate psychiatric hospitalization due to suicidal thoughts she is having. A mother who has active psychotic symptoms may need to be evaluated for medication, and a determination will need to be made about her ability to care for her children until she has stabilized. Similarly, children may be found to be at immediate risk of maltreatment. In such cases, necessary steps must be taken to ensure the safety of those involved. In difficult cases, it is best to gather as much information as possible on a parent and family before drawing conclusions about a given situation (Lieberman, 1990) and to consult with other team members or with individuals who can aid in furthering the decision process.

5

Assessing
Caregiving Capabilities

"Rock-a–Bye, Baby," the enduring lullaby of childhood, alludes simultaneously to the comforting safety and deep-seated fears of childhood. In the lullaby, a cradle and bough are depicted as environments that provide vital supports to the child. The cradle holds the child safely, while the bough protects the child from danger by bending to the winds and lulling the child to sleep. At the same time, the lullaby depicts potential dangers lurking in the background. If the winds are too strong, for instance, the bough can break, placing the child at risk.

Translated into attachment and ecological theories, the lullaby portrays a child's fundamental dependence on a caregiver for emotional nurturance, protection, and safety. The child's attachment figure, usually the parent, is the person who protects the child, keeping him or her safe from harm (Bowlby, 1988). This person ensures that the child has food and shelter and is given the love, attention, and emotional support needed to survive.

It follows that a central part of a parenting assessment involves establishing what the skills are that a mother brings to the parenting role. This chapter addresses this topic. It first introduces readers to the continuum of parenting and then describes the domains of parenting that comprise a caregiving assessment. Following this, the chapter outlines how clinicians can assess a mother's skills as a parent, how they can determine whether a mother can sustain good enough parenting over time, and how they can establish whether a mother is likely to respond to interventions.

DETERMINING WHICH STANDARD TO EVALUATE

Parenting can be conceptualized on a continuum ranging from very good parenting to at-risk and dangerous parenting (see Figure 5.1; Kempe & Kempe, 1978). Mothers who fall at the upper end of the continuum are able to meet their children's needs in an empathic, sensitive, and competent manner. Mothers whose skills as a caregiver fall at this end of the continuum are not perfect as parents. Rather, they are able to

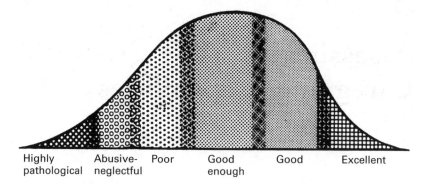

| Highly | Abusive- | Poor | Good | Good | Excellent |
| pathological | neglectful | | enough | | |

Figure 5.1.   The continuum of parenting. (From Kempe, R.S., & Kempe, H. [1978]. Cambridge, MA: Harvard University Press; adapted by permission.)

Accept [a child's] love, tolerate his demands and failings, share his pain and pleasure and get satisfaction from doing so. They may be sorely tried at times, but more than anyone else they are able to tolerate his growing pains. The child knows he is special to them, whether he is pleasing or not, well or ill, succeeding or failing. He unhesitatingly turns to them with his pleasure and miseries, confident that they will be there. He knows they are likely to see his point of view and give him the benefit of doubt before voicing critical comment. They become the brick wall he can safely kick against. Impatient or angry though they may sometimes be, he recognizes that these are often signs of their concern for him. His feelings about himself reflect his parents' feelings about him. The child whose parents value him values himself. Parents usually carry these strong feelings throughout their lives—the love, the anxiety for their children's welfare and happiness. (Winnicott, 1949, as cited in Robertson & Robertson, 1982, p. 122)

At mid-spectrum on the continuum, mothers are likely to have difficulties in consistently meeting their children's needs. A mother, for instance, may be experiencing high levels of stress, or the quality of her parenting skills may fluctuate over time. As a result, she may struggle to tolerate her child's demands and failings or experience frustration in the parenting role. Her children are not at serious risk of harm; however, neither are they being neglected or abused. Still, because her parenting is lacking in important aspects, it has a notable effect on the children's well-being.

The lower end of the parenting continuum encompasses inept or inappropriate parenting as well as poor to dangerous parenting. Mothers whose skills fall in the lower ranges of the scale do not have good enough parenting skills. Some are highly prone to stress and, in these circumstances, have serious difficulties in meeting their children's needs. Others are at risk for harming their children especially when they are overcritical of the child, have strict demands, and are feeling overwhelmed. The lowest end of the scale encompasses the parenting skills of mothers who have either placed their children in harm's way or have seriously abused or neglected them.

The first question to ask in assessing a mother's caregiving skills, then, regards the standard of parenting that is under scrutiny: Is the task to determine whether the mother meets minimal parenting standards and whether she could pose imminent risks to the child's safety and well-being, or is the clinician being asked to determine the quality of parenting skills and what issues she struggles with so as to target such areas in therapy?

Determining which standard of parenting to assess is a difficult task. For one, it can be challenging to find appropriate measures that distinguish the standard of parenting under scrutiny, especially if the issue is to determine when a parent is at risk for child maltreatment. Many measures of parenting were designed to assess the upper ends of the parenting spectrum. Moreover, standards of what constitutes *minimal* or *good enough* vary in different settings and cultures (Budd & Holdsworth, 1996). Although in many cases there is agreement about what constitutes risk or harm to a child, assessors, too, can harbor their own subjective views about what constitutes minimal or good enough parenting skills.

STARTING WITH THE PAST

Inquiring into a mother's past parenting skills, including her decision to become a parent, is a good way to begin the caregiving assessment. The following question can help frame this issue for a parent: Could you tell me about you as a parent, starting back when you became pregnant with your first child? In this context, the clinician can find out how old the mother was when she first became pregnant, whether her pregnancy was planned, how many children she has had, what the spacing was between children, whether there were long stretches of the mother's life where she was able to safely care for her children, and what factors facilitated her ability to care for her children (Zuravin, 1991).

Starting with the past helps an assessor to elucidate the specific conditions and circumstances that have contributed to a mother coming to the attention of mental health, child welfare, or legal professionals. With this information in hand, the assessor can begin constructing a trajectory of parenting that will allow for a comparison between past and present parenting skills. Obtaining baseline information on a mother's parenting skills at different points in time improves predictability. It can also indicate whether a mother's parenting has changed over time and, if so, which direction the parenting trajectory has taken.

Exploring when parenting first broke down and how serious or chronic problems have been since that time is essential for mapping out a parenting trajectory. The following questions can help clinicians to articulate these issues:

Have repeated calls been made in the past to Child Protective Services or others about the children's safety?

How long have family members been concerned about the parent or about the children in the family?

If a child was harmed or neglected in the past, how serious were the incidents?

Understanding contextual factors that have exacerbated or ameliorated a mother's difficulties in caring for her children in the past will help to clarify whether the difficulties are situational, remediable, or more serious and long-lasting.

Information on past parenting can be obtained from different sources. Mothers can be asked directly in an interview about past parenting. Probing into the past can be a delicate task, however, as it may involve delving into past trauma and into emotionally painful topics.

Talking with older children in a family can also provide rich information on past parenting. Depending on their age, some children may only be able to provide very basic descriptions about what they have experienced at home with a parent. Others may be more defensive about the assessment or worry about its outcome. Some children in these circumstances may strive to protect their parent or may place their experiences with that parent in a positive light, whereas others may be willing to express their concerns openly and provide descriptive information about experiences they have had with a parent in the past.

Clinicians should be prepared to help a child modulate feelings and to assuage fears of talking openly about family experiences if these are triggered. If inquiry is made into traumatic experiences, efforts should be taken to protect the child against unnecessary exposure to painful trauma (Lieberman & Van Horn, 2005). Very young children may not yet have the language skills to talk in depth about particular experiences. Some may not report facts accurately or may have difficulties in articulating the larger framework in which events occurred. Paying close attention to what a child says and checking this information against other sources can help a clinician to better understand the import of a young child's statements.

Relevant records (e.g., pediatric, mental health, school, child welfare) provide another important source of information on how an individual has parented in the past. Reports from Child Protective Services usually include detailed descriptions of the allegations that led the state to become involved with the family. Many reports use broad semantic categories to describe parenting qualities (e.g., poor, neglectful, abusive). As a rule of thumb, broad semantic descriptions are not useful without examining concrete examples of how a parent has cared for a child on specific occasions. Semantic descriptions are problematic because a broad range of behaviors can fall under such categories. Moreover, people may use such categories to mean different things.

Talking with family members, friends, or others (e.g., therapists, pastors, neighbors) who knew a mother at an earlier period in her life can provide additional information about past parenting if the mother gives formal permission to obtain such information. The person being interviewed should also have a clear understanding about why he or she is being contacted.

Family members may be hesitant to reveal much about a relative's parenting, especially if they believe that their statements could jeopardize reunification plans or limit contact with the child. Relatives are sometimes more prone to talk openly about their experiences if they understand that the issue is child safety and that the interviewer could help the parent and child to obtain needed interventions. At the end of an interview, it is often useful if the evaluating clinician can summarize what he or she has understood and whether it is all right to include this information in a report.

DOMAINS OF PARENTING TO ASSESS

After assessors have a grasp on a mother's past parenting skills, they can turn to what is known about the current skills that a mother brings to the parenting role. Table 5.1 provides an overview of critical domains of which assessors should gather information in the caregiving assessment.

Ability to Care for Self and Others

It is important to assess to what extent the mother can provide for herself and meet her own needs, especially if the mother's illness is chronic and severe. This includes determining whether a mother is able to maintain adequate housing for the child, hold down a job, or have enough income to make ends meet and whether she is able to get meals for herself and to provide for her own need for safety. If a mother cannot meet her own needs for shelter, safety, and food, it is highly unlikely that she will be able to provide for her children. Sorting out whether the difficulties are due to poverty alone, or to seriously compromised adaptive living skills, is essential.

Scales of adaptive living, such as the Vineland Adaptive Behavior Scales, Second Edition (Sparrow, Balla, & Cicchetti, 2005), use a structured questionnaire format to obtain objective information on a mother's overall level of adaptive functioning in various domains, including communication skills, daily living skills, socialization skills, motor skills, and maladaptive behavior.

Table 5.1. Domains of parenting

Ability to care for self and others

Is the mother able to maintain adequate housing?

Can the mother hold down a job and bring in enough income to make ends meet?

Can the mother prepare meals and obtain what she needs for living?

Can the mother ensure her own safety?

Can the mother meet her child's needs for food, shelter, clothing, and safety?

Can the mother ensure that her child is healthy?

Can the mother make sure that her child attends school?

Mother's caregiving behavior

What is the mother's ability to comfort and care for her child when he or she is ill, hurt, or frightened?

To what extent does the mother monitor her child's whereabouts?

How sensitive is the mother to her child's cues and needs?

Is the mother's discipline overly harsh or punitive?

Can the mother prioritize her child's needs?

Can the mother sustain good enough parenting over time?

Mother's understanding of child-rearing practices and development

What is the mother's understanding of development and child rearing?

What disciplinary measures does the mother endorse and enforce?

Is the mother able to flexibly change her discipline techniques depending on her children's ages and needs?

How does the mother conceptualize her role as a parent?

How does the mother feel about herself as a parent?

Mother's internal representations of child as an individual

What is the mother's understanding of her relationship with the child?

What is the mother's understanding of what her child is like as an individual?

Is the mother empathic to the child's needs?

Is the mother overly critical of the child or overly involved in his or her well-being?

Maternal coping skills

How does the mother respond to the stresses of being a parent?

How does the mother relate to others?

Is the mother impulsive in how she copes, or is she able to delay gratification?

Attachment influences

What is the mother's current state of mind about attachment?

Has the mother experienced past trauma, loss, or abuse that is affecting her parenting ability?

Did the mother experience considerable discord, control, indifference, or antipathy in her family of origin?

If a mother is unwilling or unable to provide pertinent information on self-help skills, this information can usually be obtained by interviewing individuals (e.g., family members, service coordinators, clinicians) who know the mother well. Prior permission to interview should be obtained.

Closely linked to a mother's ability to care for her own basic needs is her ability to meet her children's basic needs, including their needs for food, shelter, clothing, and safety. Other basic abilities to assess include whether the mother can ensure that her children's health and educational needs are met (see Appendix A).

Parenting Behavior

Observing how a mother interacts with her children is another essential part of the caregiving assessment (Barnum, 1997; Budd & Holdsworth, 1996; Reder & Lucey, 1995b). Observations can provide direct evidence of a mother's ability to protect her children and to supervise their whereabouts. The following features of parenting behavior are especially valuable to assess because they reveal information about the parent–child attachment relationship (Bowlby, 1988): how a mother comforts her child when the child is ill, hurt, or frightened; how she reads and responds to her children's cues; whether and how she prioritizes her children's needs; and whether she values the child and helps the child to feel safe and secure.

Questionnaires are another way that clinicians can assess parenting behavior. Because many measures have questions that ask a mother to report on her own behavior, they may have limited validity, especially if the mother is seeking to regain custody of a child. The validity of questionnaires is improved if they are part of an integrative assessment that examines patterns across data sources and time periods.

Rating scales that are based on independent observations of behavior are preferable to self-report measures because they provide a more objective measure of parenting behavior. Rating scales that have proven reliability and validity (i.e., those that can be replicated and measure what they purport to measure) should be selected whenever possible. Scales that are selected should also provide a representative sample of the parent's behavior and not just a narrow aspect of the parent's activities or attitudes (Jordan & Franklin, 2003). Clinicians should check information from rating scales with information from other sources to determine if the behavior and findings are characteristic of the parent's behavior in other settings.

Several rating scales can provide rich information on the quality of parent–child interactions. Standard rating scales, such as the Home Observation for Measurement of the Environment (HOME) inventory (Caldwell & Bradley, 2001), for instance, can help clinicians to identify at-risk parenting behavior (see also Chapter 8 and Appendix A). This measure has been used with high-risk populations (Totsika & Sylva, 2004) and can be used for a variety of age levels. Direct observational systems can provide information on parental discipline in the home (Forehand, Wells, & Griest, 1980; Reid, 1978), clinic, or laboratory (Kochanska, Kuczynski, Radke-Yarrow, & Darby-Welsh, 1987). Clinicians should keep in mind that many measures require specialized training and reliability before they can be used. Other issues to consider in deciding which tools to use are the time and cost it takes to code behavior and how well the tool distinguishes the standard of parenting under scrutiny.

Records (e.g., mental health, school, child welfare) and interviews with collateral historians who are familiar with the child and family can provide rich information about parenting behavior beyond what is observed from direct observations and questionnaires. Information on parenting behavior can also be gleaned from interviews with others familiar with the family, including neighbors and relatives. In each case, permission should be obtained before reviewing records or interviewing collateral historians about a child and parent.

Clinicians should be alert to situational influences as they interpret parenting behavior. For instance, a parent and child's behavior can change profoundly during prolonged separations (Clyman, Harden, & Little, 2002; Heinicke & Westheimer, 1965). In such instances, the interpretation of parent–child interactions will turn on several factors: the current age of the child, when the child was removed from his or her parent's care, the nature of the parent–child relationship prior to and after the separation, the regularity of parent–child visits and their quality, the child's experiences with substitute caregivers, and the attitude of substitute caregivers toward the child and toward visits (Jacobsen & Miller, 1998b).

Understanding Child Rearing and Development

A child would be at considerable risk if a mother lacked the most basic sense of what can be expected of a child at different ages. A young infant, for instance, needs to have his or her head supported in the early months of life. Similarly, toddlers can tumble down stairs or wander outside unless necessary precautions are taken in a timely manner. If a mother does not see an older child as having a need to grow up, he or she may curtail independence during middle childhood and adolescence or expect the child to provide too much care for others in the family. To successfully raise a child, then, a mother needs to have a basic understanding of child-rearing practices and of child development.

In inquiring into a mother's understanding of child rearing and development, clinicians should determine whether the mother uses excessive discipline or whether her disciplinary responses are age-appropriate and measured. In addition, they should assess how she responds to the stresses of parenting (Abidin, 1990) and whether she is able to alter her caregiving abilities in a flexible manner so as to meet the changing needs of her children as they grow older.

Paper and pencil measures can provide rich information on a mother's cognitive understanding of child-rearing techniques (Azar, Robinson, Hekimian, & Twentyman, 1984; Bavolek, 1987; Bavolek, Kline, & McLaughlin, 1979) and disciplinary measures that she endorses (Arnold, O'Leary, Wolff, & Acker, 1993). Structured interview formats can be used to identify counterproductive discipline practices (Forehand & McMahon, 1981; Patterson, Reid, Jones, & Conger, 1975; Webster-Stratton & Spitzer, 1991).

Mother's Internal Representations of Child

Attachment theorists place particular emphasis on a parent's internal representation of a child as playing an important role in influencing caregiving quality (Bowlby, 1988; Solomon & George, 1996). Mothers who can see a child's individual needs and strengths are likely to be more sensitive in meeting their needs than a mother whose understanding of the child is either highly idealized or negative (Bowlby, 1988). Part of a parent's internal representation of a child includes his or her empathy for the child and his or her ability to see his or her own needs as separate from the child's needs.

Several measures can provide rich information on a parent's internal representations of the child and on the nature of the parent's relationship to the child (George & Solomon, 1996; Zeanah, Mammen, & Lieberman, 1993). Usually, the measures ask the parent to describe the child's characteristics as well as the nature of the parent–child relationship. These interviews also inquire into whether the parent planned for this child, how she felt about the child at birth, how she chose the child's name and why, and how the relationship has changed or evolved over time.

A measure of expressed emotion (Magana et al., 1986; Magana-Amato, 1993) can supplement the information on a mother's internal working model by articulating aspects of dysfunctional parenting. This measure specifically establishes whether the parent is overly critical or overly involved in a specific child or relationship. High expressed emotion (e.g., an overly critical and/or overly involved relationship) has been associated with family conflict at home (Hibbs, Hamburger, Kruesi, & Lenane, 1993), marital difficulties, parental coldness toward a child (Stubbe, Zahner, Goldstein, & Leckman, 1993), disorganized attachment status in children (Jacobsen, Hibbs, & Ziegenhain, 2000), and symptom exacerbation in children of different ages (Hibbs et al.,

1991; Schwartz, Dorer, Beardslee, Lavori, & Keller, 1990; Stubbe et al., 1993).

Some mothers may be reluctant to reveal ambivalent feelings about a child in an assessment. This is sometimes the case in very young mothers or in mothers who have had a child under traumatic experiences. Family and societal pressures may contribute to these mothers insisting that they have only positive feelings toward a specific child. Getting at ambivalence in such cases can often be challenging and difficult. Sometimes this information is only revealed by a mother later on. One mother, for instance, insisted that she wanted to regain custody of both of her children. However, she consistently spent more time with her younger child. Her interactions with the younger child were also more positive and rewarding. The mother revealed only much later that the child she spent little time with was conceived from the man who raped her.

Personality Influences

Several characteristics of a mother's personality have been associated with risk for child maltreatment. Poor impulse control, difficulties in relating to and confiding in others, and difficulties in verbalizing one's feelings about children, for instance, have been linked to risk for child neglect (Gaudin, Polansky, & Kilpatrick, 1992). Chronic coping difficulties, a chronic sense of hopelessness, deep-seated deficits in caring for children in the past, poor coping skills, and poor problem-solving abilities are factors that have been shown to bode poorly for future parenting (Adshead, Falkov, & Göpfert, 2004). These areas are another aspect of parenting capacity to assess.

Attachment Influences

Experiences of abuse, neglect, trauma, loss, or major separations make a parent more vulnerable to maltreatment, although they do not, in themselves, determine whether a mother will abuse or neglect her children (Bowlby, 1988). Some parents who were maltreated in childhood may struggle in prioritizing their children's needs especially if they as parents are under stress. In such situations, a mother may turn to her children for comfort or help or may abdicate the parenting role until her own stress and emotional needs are assuaged (Solomon & George, 1996).

Inquiring into the childhood experiences of a mother is, therefore, an important part of the caregiving assessment. The Life Events and Difficulties Scale (Bifulco, Brown, & Harris, 1994) is one measure that can be used to assess a mother's childhood experiences. This measure provides information on a mother's quality of relationships with parenting in childhood, past trauma, the consequences of loss of a parent in childhood, discord in the home, physical and sexual abuse, as well as parental indifference and parental control and antipathy.

The Adult Attachment Interview (AAI; George & Main, 1984) provides rich information on a parent's current state of mind about attachment relationships, both past and present. In evaluating the AAI, the clinician first reviews critical experiences that could influence parenting (e.g., loss of caregiver, witnessing violence, disruptions in care, positive experiences, support) and looks for major contradictions from other sources and reports. The assessor then reviews what the mother says about her caregivers (e.g., "great," "cruel," "abusive") and examines the fit between her descriptions and the evidence (or lack of it) she provides to support the descriptions. Other parts of the evaluation look at how coherent the mother's account of her childhood attachment experiences are, whether she values attachment relationships, and whether she can see how attachment experiences in childhood have affected her own development, including her parenting of her own children. The following types of questions can help an evaluator to elucidate these effects: Does the mother acknowledge that past attachment experiences exert an effect on who she is today? Does she focus only on positive experiences at the expense of negative experiences? Does the mother state that she wants to do things differently from what she experienced in childhood?

The AAI distinguishes a mother's state of mind about attachment. Four groups are distinguished: dismissive, preoccupied, unresolved, and autonomous (Hesse, 1999). Parents who dismiss past effects are more likely to repeat problems from the past, especially if caregivers are idealized. They may be less prone to read and respond to their child's distress and may reject the child at vulnerable moments. A mother who is preoccupied with past experiences may be at a higher risk for experiencing separation anxiety; have difficulties reading the child's cues, especially if she is preoccupied with her own thoughts; and strongly rely on a child to meet his or her own attachment needs. Mothers who are unresolved about the past are likely to repeat past mistakes because they are not aware of the effects of the past. Mothers with an autonomous state of mind value attachment experiences, but recognize the effects on the self.

Not surprisingly, the autonomous state of mind is most typically associated with secure attachment in children. Such mothers are comfortable with their own and with their children's attachment needs. The dismissive, preoccupied, and unresolved states of mind are associated with insecure child–parent attachment patterns. Although providing rich clinical information on adult states of mind regarding attachment (Sagi et al., 1994), the AAI takes considerable training, and the classification process is time consuming.

The Attachment Style Interview (ASI) inquires into an individual's support network and how he or she relates to his or her partner or romantic relationship (Bifulco, Moran, Ball, & Bernazzani, 2002). Questions are asked to obtain information on how much the informant confides in his or her partner, how much active emotional support the partner gives, and the quality of interaction. Inquiries are also made into the parent's experiences with caregivers in his or her family of origin and his or her relationship with friends and siblings. A classification system also rates parents as enmeshed, dismissive, fearful, or withdrawn. A standard category is used for mothers who have a good ability to make and maintain attachment relationships. The ASI requires training, but it can be scored relatively quickly. It provides valuable information on a parent's ability to establish and maintain supportive relationships.

SUSTAINING PARENTING SKILLS

How a parent responds over the course of a one- or two-hour observation can reveal important information about caregiving. A clinician will, nonetheless, need to establish whether the parent can sustain good enough or at least minimal parenting skills over time. Observing a mother in different settings with her children and obtaining information on how she deals with her children over longer periods of time, especially in times of stress, can help an assessor get a handle on this issue. Information on a mother's ability to sustain parenting over time can also be obtained through interviewing people familiar with the parent and by conducting longer observations.

THE ISSUE OF CHANGE

Many individuals who have evidenced serious breakdown in parenting are able to change problematic aspects of their parenting to safely raise their children (Jacobsen & Miller, 1998b). For others, change takes place slowly and not in a time frame that makes sense for the child (Goldstein et al., 1998). Because of differences in rates of change, if a mother poses risks to her children, then it is important to determine her potential to change her parenting skills in a time frame that makes sense for her children. The following list of questions provides a framework for clinicians to use in determining this issue:

1. Is the individual highly motivated to change her parenting?

2. Is she able to assume responsibility for past problems she has had in parenting her children?

3. Has she actively sought out help to address her parenting problems?

4. Has she established solid working alliances with others?

5. Is she able to respond to feedback about her parenting skills?

6. Are there signs that she is internalizing change?

7. Is she able to establish and maintain supportive relationships?

CULTURAL INFLUENCES

Parents who come from different cultural and ethnic backgrounds have their own unique ways of caring for and raising their children. These practices may vary greatly from what is accepted in the United States and with what an assessor may be familiar. Although a clinician cannot know everything about parenting and child rearing in all cultures, reading about parenting in other cultures can greatly expand understanding and aid in an assessment. Asking parents about their culture shows an interest in learning. When asked, families are usually open and willing to explain cultural and family practices and to tell an assessor their views on raising children.

Difficulties can, nonetheless, arise if the way a mother raises her child is seen by her as legitimate, but if this way is viewed by clinicians and others as harming the child or placing him or her at risk. In approaching such issues, Lieberman (1989) suggested that clinicians should start by learning more about the child-rearing practices in question. In this process, they should maintain an attitude of openness to understand all they can about the practice and its meaning for the family. The following case illustrates just how important an attitude of openness can be.

Elena had her toddler removed from her care following allegations that she had kept him in a cardboard box for long periods of time. Elena had been living in the United States for only one year. She had few economic resources and always lived on the edge of poverty. An assessment revealed that she, indeed, did keep her son in a cardboard box, but when the practice was explored, Elena explained that she used the box as a playpen when she cooked. She had no funds to purchase a real playpen and could better monitor her son's whereabouts during meal preparation.

If there is clear evidence of abuse or neglect, then clinicians will need to take issue with the mother's child-rearing practices. To ensure children's safety, mental health professionals are mandated reporters and are required by law to report abusive or neglectful parenting to child welfare authorities. Clinicians need to remind parents of this duty to report in a calm, thoughtful, and nonthreatening manner. Focus should be placed on maintaining the therapeutic alliance (Lieberman, 1990).

IS THE CHILD AT RISK?

The information gathered during the caregiving assessment provides the foundation for determining whether children in the family are at risk, whether the problems that are identified can truly be considered to be serious (Herbert & Harper-Dorton, 2002). Mental health professionals should be careful that the results of an assessment show reasonable cause to suspect that the child is suffering or is likely to suffer significant harm (Herbert & Harper-Dorton, 2002). In this determination, it is important to consider the likely effects on the child if the situation does not improve and to consider the likelihood of change in the parent.

Part of assessing risk involves determining whether there is a sufficient fit between a child and his or her mother (Goldstein et al., 1998; Göpfert, Webster, & Nelki, 2004b, p. 96). For instance, a mother who has one child with autism and another with no delays will need to be evaluated on a higher standard for the child with special needs. Assessing the question of fit will require looking at what is known about parenting in relation to what is known about the child's history and his or her individual needs and well-being. What is important is that the fit between child and parent is good enough for the particular child and in the particular circumstances in which the family lives.

Determining how serious the risk to a child is can be a complex endeavor, and clinicians should be familiar with definitions and descriptions of what constitutes child abuse and neglect. In many cases, the level of risk posed by a parent may involve emotional abuse or neglect. The following are parental behaviors and attitudes that constitute emotional risk (Adshead et al., 2004; Bowlby, 1988; Lieberman, 1993):

- Persistent rejection or scapegoating of a child

- Frequent ridiculing or dismissing the child's fears

- Ongoing threats to abandon the child

- Persistently failing to recognize the child's individual needs

- Repeatedly blaming the child for how the parent feels

- Being persistently critical of the child

- Curbing or restricting the child's interests and mobility to meet the needs of the parent

- Evidence that the parent does not love the child

- Consistently favoring one child over another in the family

- Failing to provide praise or encouragement to the child

- Highly inappropriate expectations of the child

- Being emotionally unavailable to the child

- Expecting the child to care for the mother or for siblings to the extent that the child's needs are seriously neglected

Several assessment tools are available that can help identify parents most at risk for serious parenting problems. The Child Well Being Scales (Magura & Moses, 1986), the Child Abuse Potential Inventory (Milner, 1980), the Ontario Child Neglect Index (Trocme, 1996), and the Childhood Level of Living Scale (Polansky, Cabral, Magura, & Phillips, 1983; Polansky, Chalmers, Buttenweiser, & Williams, 1978) are some common instruments used to assess the extent and nature of maltreatment by a parent that a child may be experiencing in a home. References listed in Appendix B may also help clinicians to recognize and understand the various forms of child maltreatment, especially in complex cases.

As underscored earlier, notions of what constitutes child abuse and neglect are not always clear cut. They can vary greatly across settings and cultures and even across assessors on the same team (Lieberman, 1989). In some cases, the issue of harm and detriment to a child's well-being may be clear cut and easily definable for all involved. Unfortunately, this is not always the case.

When the consequences of parenting behavior for a child's well-being are unclear or ambiguous, it may be difficult to establish whether the harm to a child is significant enough to report. In such cases, clinicians should not rush to judgment until they have a full understanding of the parent's behaviors and of what happened. If after knowing more it becomes clear that the issues are serious, swift and appropriate action should be taken to ensure the safety of the child (Lieberman, 1989).

6

The Psychiatric Evaluation

The psychiatric evaluation provides the clinician with information on the nature and type of the symptoms the parent is exhibiting, whether the parent has a diagnosable psychiatric disorder and, if so, what the disorder is, what the prognosis of the disorder is, what its longitudinal course is likely to look like, and what interventions can make a difference.

This information is critical for a larger parenting assessment. It is a prerequisite for answering the question of whether an individual's illness symptoms are having an impact on his or her abilities to parent. A psychiatric evaluation could reveal that a parent does not have a mental illness or that she was misdiagnosed. In some cases, a parent may have been given only a provisional psychiatric diagnosis due to a lack of available information at the time of the assessment. In such cases, a comprehensive psychiatric evaluation can clarify, confirm, or reject a diagnosis. If a parent does have a diagnosable psychiatric disorder, the diagnostic picture helps the clinician to establish an optimal treatment plan.

This chapter describes the psychiatric evaluation, including the psychiatric interview, and the mental status examination (MSE). It then discusses how diagnoses are formulated and how a psychiatric evaluation is conducted when it is undertaken in the context of a larger parenting assessment. Next, the chapter looks at the structure of the report and considers what clinicians can do to gather sound information on how a mother's psychiatric symptoms may affect her ability to care for her children. The chapter concludes by discussing psychiatric considerations to keep in mind when assessing parenting risk during pregnancy and in the postpartum period.

For psychiatrists, this chapter underscores what is unique and essential about a psychiatric evaluation undertaken in the context of a parenting assessment. For those mental health, child welfare, or legal professionals who work with mothers with psychiatric diagnoses but who are not psychiatrists, the chapter provides a framework for understanding how a psychiatric evaluation can be meaningfully used in the context of a larger assessment of parenting. Although they may not conduct such evaluations, assessors should understand the purpose and scope of a psychiatric evaluation.

THE PSYCHIATRIC EVALUATION

In a comprehensive medical psychiatric evaluation, the clinician interviews the parent to obtain a full biopsychosocial history. The clinician also performs an MSE; speaks with collateral historians who have treated or are treating the parent; orders any additional medical tests; and requests relevant medical, psychiatric, psychological, or criminal records. Neurological or other medical tests (e.g., a brain scan) may be needed if symptoms are present, if the parent's history suggests a regression in cognitive or physical functioning, or if there is the possibility of brain injury or seizures.

In obtaining a complete history from the parent and in formulating the psychiatric diagnosis, the clinician elicits and integrates data from various sources (see Table 6.1).

Psychiatric Interview

During the individual interview, the clinician elicits information about the parent's background (e.g., age, ethnicity, marital status, employment, number of children) and her perspective of her medical history and symptoms, including the history of her illness, its onset, symptom exacerbations, periods of stability, hospitalizations, and her history and pattern of using substances. In this context, questions are asked about suicide attempts, arrests, and any other dangerous or self-destructive behavior. The clinician also inquires into the parent's past and current psychiatric treatment and gathers documentation on which treatment venues (e.g., day programs, medications, therapy, partial

Table 6.1. Sources used in the psychiatric evaluation

Individual interview

Mental status examination

Observations of parent during interview

Review of records
    Past psychiatric records: inpatient and outpatient
    Substance abuse evaluations
    Relevant medical records
    Past psychological evaluations
    Child welfare records
    Therapist reports
    Criminal background records

Interviews with collateral historians
    Mental health professionals providing care to mother
    Family members
    Service coordinator

hospitalizations) the parent has rejected or accepted. Obtaining information on the parent's response to treatment is part of the interview.

Mental Status Examination

The Mental Status Examination (MSE)—a key component of a standard medical psychiatric evaluation—inquires into auditory and visual hallucinations and gathers information on how the parent relates to the evaluator, the most important themes that the parent brings up, how organized and coherent the parent's thought processes are, her insight and judgment, and the extent to which she accepts responsibility for her mental illness and other problems (Miller et al., 1998). Data on a parent's defense mechanisms (e.g., denial, intellectualization) and particularly sensitive subjects or issues that may need to be addressed in therapy are also gathered in this examination based on a parent's responses to interview questions and on observations of nonverbal behavior.

The Diagnosis

Integrating information from the various parts of the psychiatric interview and from the various sources (e.g., record reviews, interviews with collateral historians) provides the basis for the psychiatric diagnosis. In formulating a diagnosis, the psychiatrist pays particular attention to a mother's symptoms, their etiology and course, and their overall patterning. In making the diagnosis, the psychiatrist relies on the *DSM-IV-TR* (American Psychiatric Association, 2000). This manual elucidates the criteria used to make psychiatric diagnoses and to assess the individual's functioning across five main axes:

Axis I: Clinical disorders

Axis II: Personality disorders and mental retardation

Axis III: General medical conditions

Axis IV: Psychosocial and environmental problems

Axis V: Global assessment of functioning

In addition to providing a standard framework for assessing an individual's functioning across the above five axes, the *DSM-IV-TR* includes severity (i.e., mild, moderate, severe) and course specifiers that mark whether the illness is in full or partial remission. Provisional diagnoses can also be used if there is a strong presumption that the full criteria may ultimately be met for a specific disorder, although there is currently not enough available information to make a firm diagnosis (American Psychiatric Association, 2000).

When the Evaluation Is Part of a Parenting Assessment

A psychiatric evaluation that is undertaken as part of a larger parenting assessment gathers the same information that is obtained for the standard medical psychiatric evaluation. However, information on parenting is also systematically gathered, considered, and integrated into the assessment.

Answers to three overarching questions should be ascertained in this evaluation:

1. Do the mother's mental illness symptoms place her child at an increased risk for maltreatment or harm?

2. Are there longer-term effects of the mother's mental illness symptoms on the child's well-being that need to be considered in developing a treatment plan?

3. If the mother's current treatment plan is changed, will it likely bring about an improvement in her parenting skills?

Asking about a mother's medical and psychosocial history provides a port of entry for finding out about her parenting. How many pregnancies has a mother had? Were they planned? How did she feel about each pregnancy? How has the mother's mental illness symptoms affected her parenting? When is she best able to parent? When does she struggle? What are her weaknesses and strengths as a parent?

The overall goal is to map out points of intersection between a mother's parenting trajectory in relation to the onset, history, and course of her mental illness. Key questions to keep in mind while mapping out the two trajectories and discerning how they relate to each other include the following:

1. What is parenting like when the mother is operating at her best (e.g., when her illness is in remission or stabilized)?

2. What is parenting like when the mother has episodes of active psychiatric symptoms (e.g., hallucinations, depression)?

3. What factors exacerbate her illness?

4. What is the overall prognosis for the mother's illness?

5. Is it likely that if the mother responds to treatment, her parenting will change for the better?

6. What is the likelihood that a mother will stick to a helpful treatment regimen?

The construction of a timeline that examines the mother's symptoms and psychiatric history (e.g., hospitalizations) in relation to parenting events (e.g., births of children, custody loss) and changes in the family and environment (e.g., separation, loss, divorce) can help organize a complex history.

Structure of Report

After obtaining a clear diagnostic picture and establishing whether, how, and to what extent parenting may be affected by a mother's mental illness symptoms, a formal report is composed and written. This report integrates information on parenting into the different sections of the psychiatric report.

The report will list the parent's name, the name of the evaluating psychiatrist, and the dates and locations of the interviews. After documenting what the purpose of the evaluation is and pertinent identifying data for the mother, all sources of information that were drawn on in the psychiatric evaluation will be listed. The list of sources should be specific, noting the type of report (e.g., psychiatric evaluation, psychological testing), institution or clinic, the dates when the report was written, and the assessor's name and degree(s).

In the main section of the report, data from the psychiatric interview with the parent are summarized. This section will include a discussion of the history of the parent's psychiatric illness, the parent's history of violence, suicide attempts, arrests, or other dangerous behavior, the parent's past medical history, her family's psychiatric history, her psychosocial history, and her current treatment (e.g., medications, psychosocial). The parent's history of compliance with treatment is then discussed, followed by a summary of information gathered from written records and from collateral historians. A summary of the MSE, a formulation of the diagnosis (how the diagnosis was derived, how certain the diagnosis is, and what it means), and the listing of all *DSM-IV* diagnoses follow. The final section of the report will explicitly discuss how a mother's mental illness symptoms may or have affected the mother's past and current parenting. Included at the end of the report, this section also discusses whether treatment may affect the parenting trajectory and whether the mother is likely to respond to treatment in a time frame that makes sense for her child(ren).

The following descriptions illustrate some ways that a concluding section of a psychiatric report can address issues about parenting:

Ms. Lane has received effective treatment for her psychiatric illness and is currently experiencing few symptoms. She has been capable of safely parenting her two children. Her illness does not preclude her showing good judgment and good parenting skills. However, when faced with multiple stresses, she may be vulnerable to becoming overwhelmed and having difficulty in attending to relevant cues from her children. The good alliance she has with her therapist suggests the likelihood that she would ask for help when she feels overwhelmed, which greatly decreases the risk of neglect. She would benefit from ongoing therapy and should continue her psychotropic medication.

Ms. Burns' inability to sustain effective treatment for her bipolar disorder places her at a high risk for relapse. While acutely depressed and/or manic, Ms. Burns' parenting is expected to be greatly impaired. During past episodes of depression and/or mania, she had become suicidal and violent at times. These symptoms would likely recur in future episodes unless she accepts the need for consistent treatment. Ongoing drinking of alcoholic beverages would likely increase the frequency and severity of her bipolar disorder.

OBTAINING SOUND INFORMATION

How an evaluation is undertaken can greatly have an impact on the quality of information gathered. The following sections present several hints that may aid clinicians in obtaining sound information in a psychiatric evaluation (Miller et al., 1998).

Alleviating Stress

Because parenting is an immensely important life role (Apfel & Handel, 1993), a mother will naturally be worried, frightened, angry, or unsure about a psychiatric evaluation, especially if it involves questions about her parenting capacity or if issues of custody are at stake. Acknowledging the stress directly and taking a nonjudgmental stance can alleviate some of the stress of the evaluation. Letting a mother know whether her records have been read beforehand and clarifying whether the evaluation will be confidential may also alleviate stress. Letting a mother know what your precise role is (assessor, advocate, and so forth) and reminding her how and when she will receive feedback about the evaluation can also be reassuring and can get the evaluation off to a good start.

A Focus on Symptoms

Clinicians should keep in mind that illness dimensions and symptoms may be more important predictors of parenting risk and competency than the psychiatric diagnosis per se (Kumar et al., 1995; Sameroff et al., 1982). They should, therefore, be alert to the specifics of a mother's symptoms and should know what illness dimensions and symptoms can increase parenting risk.

Table 6.2. Symptoms that may increase risk

Severity of illness symptoms
Chronicity of illness
Early age of onset of illness
Comorbid psychiatric illness
Comorbid substance use or abuse problems
Active psychotic symptoms (e.g., paranoia, delusions)
Rapidly changing mental states
Aggressive, violent, or suicidal behavior
Deteriorating judgment
Presence of command hallucinations
Child included in parent's delusions
Low insight into mental illness
Parent is not compliant with treatment
Parent is not responsive to treatment
Poor cognitive processing
Low level of adaptive functioning
History of family violence, neglect, parental substance
    abuse, or parental psychiatric disorders

Table 6.2 provides an overview of various psychiatric symptoms that can increase parenting risk (see also Göpfert, Webster, & Seeman, 2004; Jacobsen & Miller, 1998b; Reder & Lucey, 1995a).

Detailed Descriptions

In reviewing relevant mental health, child welfare, and legal records, clinicians should look for detailed descriptions of symptoms and behaviors. Descriptions, if detailed and clear, are usually far more telling of the nature of a mother's parenting and her psychiatric symptoms than are labels. Labels and evaluative terms such as *abusing, neglectful,* or *unstable* are usually too broad and too vague. Moreover, they can mean different things to different assessors. Detailed descriptions document specific behaviors, symptoms, and contexts. They are telling as they can provide accurate and useful information on the meaning of specific symptoms or behaviors.

A Longitudinal Approach

Clinicians should look at a trajectory of parenting and compare information on a mother's parenting at different points of time (see Chapter 8). A mother may have had major difficulties in parenting at one point in her life, but if these problems occurred 10 years ago and the mother's behavior has changed, this is important to know. Comparing behavior over time can reveal information about a longitudinal trajectory of parenting and changes a mother has undergone as a parent.

Learning from Discrepancies

Clinicians should note major discrepancies in the interview and address these directly by asking the parent to explain the contradictions. If the parent's explanation is logical and plausible, then contradictions may be resolved. By contrast, if a mother cannot explain the contradictions or if she becomes defiant or changes the storyline, that information is important to know, too. It can tell the assessor how believable the mother's account is, how she relates to others, what her mental status is, or what predominant defenses she is using. Keeping track of discrepancies also points to additional areas that will need further investigation.

Collateral Interviews

In talking with mental health providers who are treating or have treated a parent, clinicians should establish how long the provider has known the mother, what type of treatment he or she has offered her, what the specific goals of the treatment were, what the therapeutic alliance was like, and how long the treatment was or is expected to take.

If the provider offers information on parenting capability or risk, the clinician should clarify the source of that information. It is important to establish whether the provider is basing the estimation of risk on direct observations he has made of the mother with her children, whether this is his view, whether the observations are current, and whether the provider is an advocate for the mother.

Clarifying Information

In the process of determining whether a mother's symptoms are having an effect on child safety and well-being, clinicians should clarify anything that is confusing. For instance, if a mother reports that she heard voices or experienced an impulse to harm, it is critical to find out whether the voices or impulses ever directly involved her child. If a mother's delusions have not involved her child and if she has never acted on her delusions, the risk to parenting is likely to be substantially lower than it would be if her delusions directly implicated her child (e.g., child is seen as a "sacrificial lamb").

If a mother has an impulse to harm, it is important to clarify how the mother is experiencing the impulse. If the impulses to harm are experienced as obsessive, intrusive, and incongruent with reality, it may not lead to harmful behaviors but rather to safety checking or avoidance behaviors (e.g., repetitive checking to ensure that the child is safe) (Wisner, Peindl, Gigliotti, & Hanusa, 1999). Clarifying whether children were involved in any suicidal ideation or attempts or in other forms of violent behavior is also essential.

Contextual Influences

Clinicians should pay attention to and document contexts in the mother's history that have facilitated parenting and that have led to improvement in her mental health and functioning. If there is a high likelihood that she can maintain a supportive environment for parenting and if her illness symptoms have stabilized through treatment, the outcome will be better than the outcome of a mother who is not actively engaged in treatment and who has difficulties in maintaining a supportive environment for parenting.

A Strengths Perspective

As noted again and again, literature on parents with mental illness is focused predominately on the detrimental effects that mental illness can exert on parenting and on children (Nicholson et al., 2001). For understanding the larger picture that comprises a comprehensive assessment, however, it is also vital to look at strengths (Ackerson, 2003). Examining strengths puts a focus on what needs to be done to promote better parenting outcomes and a safe environment for children. It also opens opportunities for treatment and rehabilitation that may otherwise be missed (Nicholson et al., 2001).

Protective factors that assessors should be alert to in the psychiatric evaluation include whether the mother has a mild form of mental illness, whether she is compliant with and responds rapidly to treatment (Uddenberg & Engelsson, 1978), whether she has a viable support network that provides her with enough emotional support both as an individual and as a parent, whether she has a good therapeutic alliance with mental health professionals, whether she is motivated to learn and change, and whether she had positive role models and experiences in childhood (Fendrich, Warner, & Weissman, 1990; Lynch & Roberts, 1977).

Insight into Illness

Clinicians should pay attention to a mother's level of insight into her psychiatric illness. Good insight has been linked to better illness outcomes (McEvoy, Appelbaum, Apperson, Geller, & Freter, 1989), better adherence to psychotropic medication and psychosocial treatments (Amador, Strauss, Yale, & Gorman, 1991), and better psychosocial and vocational functioning (Lysaker,

Bell, Milstein, Bryson, & Beam-Goulet, 1994; Soskis & Bowers, 1969). Mothers with good insight into their mental illness also appear to be at a lower risk for harming their children than mothers who lack insight into their illness (Mullick et al., 2001), although an overall risk equation should include a multiplicity of factors.

Several scales are available for assessing insight into mental illness (Amador et al., 1991; David, 1990; Mullick et al., 2001). These scales rate the extent to which a parent thinks she has a mental illness, how she explains her illness (e.g., plausible mechanisms, confusion, delusion), to what extent she accepts treatment, and whether she takes initiative in requesting treatment when needed (Miller et al., 1998; Mullick et al., 2001). A mother who has little insight into her illness may fail to recognize symptoms of her illness, misattribute the source or cause of her symptoms, or fail to appreciate the implausibility of her delusions or perceptual experiences (Sackheim, 1998). A mother with good insight is aware of her symptoms, takes the initiative in seeking out treatment when needed, and understands that treatment can make a difference (Amador et al., 1991).

Assessing Potential for Change

Clinicians should establish whether a mother's condition is likely to worsen or stabilize over time and determine whether treatment will make a difference. Addressing these issues requires an understanding of the mother's past treatment regimens and how she has responded to treatment. The following questions can guide a clinician in assessing a mother's potential for change (Miller et al., 1998):

1. What is the mother's adherence to medication?

2. Is it taken regularly and then stopped when she is doing well?

3. Does the mother manage her own medication, or does a family member or service coordinator do this?

4. What is the optimal treatment plan for the mother?

5. What is the mother's adherence to the current treatment?

6. How efficacious is her current treatment plan?

7. Will the treatment be able to continue for as long as the parent needs it, or is there a limit to the length of the treatment?

Assessing the likelihood of change requires evaluating whether a mother has the capacity to benefit from treatment and if this is likely to occur. Table 6.3 lists factors that are often indicative of a more positive prognosis (Fitzpatrick, 1995; Gabbard, 2000).

Table 6.3. Likelihood of change

Strong motivation to understand and change
Ownership of illness
Ownership of own difficulties
Ability to see mental health professionals as potentially helpful
Significant suffering
Capacity for insight
A viable and meaningful support network
Tolerance for frustration
Ability to sustain a job
Ability to listen to and respond to feedback

Motivation and willpower are underestimated protective factors in many evaluations (Ghaemi, 1999). What is important to see is that a mother has the motivation to change and to work to solve parenting problems to which she has contributed. Often, this can best be assessed by observing the mother's typical pattern of response to treatment and by interviewing past and present treatment providers. What is important to sort out is if a mother is genuinely motivated to change and whether she is actively engaged in treatment or is just going through the motions to satisfy others (e.g., a child welfare agency).

ASSESSING RISK IN PREGNANCY AND IN THE POSTPARTUM PERIOD

The period around childbirth is often an especially vulnerable time for women with regard to psychiatric illness (Spinelli, 1999). Studies indicate that between 9% and 14% of women may develop clinical depression during pregnancy (O'Connor, Hawkins, Dunn, Thorpe, & Golding, 1998). Between 10% and 20% of women develop postpartum depression (Jofesson, Berg, Nordin, & Sydsjö, 2001). One in 500 to 1,000 women experience postpartum psychosis (Spinelli, 1999). If a woman has a prior history of a major mood disorder, however, she is about 300 times more likely than other women to have illness exacerbations in the postpartum period (Hamilton & Sichel, 1992).

The symptoms of a major episode of depression in pregnancy are the same as the symptoms that occur when an individual becomes clinically depressed at other phases in her life. Symptoms of depression may, nonetheless, go unrecognized because pregnancy changes can often cause similar symptoms to those seen in depression, such as increased tiredness, emotional mood changes, and weight gain.

If a mother becomes clinically depressed during pregnancy, there can be many risks both to the baby and to the mother. A mother who becomes depressed while she is pregnant may not eat well. She may lose weight and fail to seek out prenatal care for her baby. She may also increase her use of substances, including smoking and alcohol use.

Recognizing factors that increase the risk that a pregnant woman will develop depression is, therefore, important. The following are important factors that can increase risk: a past episode of depression or a history of substance abuse, a family history of mental illness, marital problems, little support, anxiety about the unborn baby, and problems with a past pregnancy or birth.

Postpartum depression occurs within 6 months of a woman giving birth to her baby. The symptoms of postpartum depression are the same as those for clinical depression seen at other periods in the life cycle. They include sleep and appetite disturbances, impaired concentration, feelings of inadequacy, and a sad or irritable mood. Sometimes these symptoms are directly related to parenting. For instance, a mother may feel that she is not a good enough parent.

The most important risk factors for postpartum depression include a previous history of major depression, especially during the antenatal period (Heron et al., 2004), a family history of mood disorder (O'Hara, Neunaber, & Zekoski, 1984; Thorpe, Golding, MacGillivray, & Greenwood, 1991), inadequate social support, and stress (O'Hara, 1986).

Postpartum depression should be distinguished from the postpartum blues, which is a typical response to birth. The blues occur in approximately 50% of women after pregnancy. Characterized by a heightened reactivity to stimuli (Miller, 2002), women with the blues are more irritable, cry more easily, and are more emotionally labile than usual. The emotions associated with the blues peak 3–5 days after delivery and may last for several days to weeks. In contrast to postpartum depression, the propensity to develop the blues is not linked to a mother's past psychiatric history or stress.

Postpartum psychosis is a rare condition that usually severely impairs a mother's ability to function (Steiner & Tam, 1999). Characterized by hallucinations and/or delusions, it has a rapid onset and typically occurs within the first few days to 2–3 weeks postpartum. Women who develop psychosis in the postpartum period may lead mental health professionals to believe that they are well but may become profoundly psychotic or depressed soon after (Miller, 2002). In rare and extreme cases, there is a high risk of infanticide or suicide, but if treated, the prognosis is usually good (Millis & Kornblith, 1992).

Both postpartum depression and psychosis can greatly affect a mother's parenting and, if untreated, may place her infant's development and attachment at considerable risk. These findings make it imperative for clinicians to identify women at the highest risk and to prevent episodes of mood disorders before they emerge. Diagnosing and treating mood disorders during pregnancy may prevent long-term damaging effects on offspring and preserve a mother's role as parent.

There are several ports of entry for assessing parenting risk during pregnancy. A clinician can ask how a mother feels about her unborn baby, whether

Table 6.4. Risk factors during pregnancy

Denial of pregnancy
Marked ambivalence about wanting the baby
Exacerbation of a pre-existing psychiatric illness during pregnancy
Delusions about baby or pregnancy
Lack of normal fantasies and beliefs about the unborn baby
Significant family tension due to anticipated change in role relationships
Thoughts of killing or harming unborn baby
Refusal of necessary prenatal care
Actions designed to kill or harm unborn baby
New onset of psychiatric illness during pregnancy
Suicide attempt during pregnancy

From personal communication, Laura J. Miller, M.D., January 20, 2001.

she is looking forward to the birth of her baby, what she thinks the baby will be like, whether she has made concrete plans about the delivery and what will happen afterward, and whether she has chosen a name for the baby. Mothers who have given no thought to the infant's name or who have a highly negative attitude toward the birth are likely to have increased parenting problems postpartum (Crittenden & Morrison, 1988; Righetti-Veltema, Bousquet, & Manzano, 2003). Several other red flags for identifying mothers at the most risk for parenting problems when they are pregnant are listed in Table 6.4.

If a mother becomes severely depressed after childbirth or develops other significant psychiatric symptoms, a parenting assessment can allow for optimal treatment to ensure a baby's safety and to benefit the developing parent–infant relationship. Being aware of factors that may indicate difficulties in the early mother–infant attachment relationship is critical. Some risk factors for serious parenting problems in the postnatal period are listed in Table 6.5.

Table 6.5. Risk factors in the postpartum period

Obsessional thoughts and complaints, especially concerning the baby. Be alert especially to somatic preoccupations.
Hostility toward the baby, husband, and those who are close to the parent.
Apathy to the baby and indifference to caregiving instruction.
Anxiety that produces excessive questioning about the same thing repeatedly.
Failure to bond in the first 3 days of life.
Difficulty responding appropriately to the baby's basic needs.
Projections of adult feelings onto the infant (e.g., "Look how angry he is at me!").
Neglect of basic baby care, such as feeding, diaper changing, and dressing of the baby.
Difficulty talking with the baby and/or maintaining eye contact and a conversation, even with a young baby.

From Apfel, R.J., & Handel, M.H. (1993). Madness and loss of motherhood: Sexuality, reproduction, and long-term mental illness. Arlington, VA: American Psychiatric Press; adapted by permission.

7

Social and Environmental Influences

Heather Hasslinger

How parents with serious mental illness interact with the environment can proffer both protective and risk factors for themselves and their children. Parents who can provide a safe home environment, establish and maintain a network of supportive relationships, and obtain necessary services for themselves and their children are likely to fare better in the parenting role than parents who have difficulties with these tasks (Jacobsen et al., 1997). From a social work perspective, when a parent suffers from a serious mental illness, the parent can have greater challenges in adapting to and managing surrounding social and environmental stressors, and young children can be at an increased developmental risk. For this reason, this chapter views families within an ecological framework (Mattaini & Meyer, 2002) that accounts for familial strengths and limitations, social supports and stresses, and environmental resources and pressures (Germain & Bloom, 1999). Clinicians can structure their parenting assessment by assessing the quality of a parent's transactions with three levels of the environment: the home setting (micro-system), the parent's support network within and outside of her family (mezzo-system), and the larger community and societal factors that can have an impact on parenting (macro-system).

Experienced clinicians also recognize that patterns of behavior that parents exhibit in interacting with their environment and with their children can be, in part, determined by parents' past attachment experiences. Although not inevitable, parents who have suffered childhood neglect and/or abuse can unwittingly repeat their own childhood experiences with their children. For this reason, this chapter also utilizes an attachment perspective (Bowlby, 1988) to aid assessors in making perfunctory assessments of the quality of parent–child interactions and in recognizing when repetition of abuse and neglect is more or less likely (Hesse, 1999).

Last, in approaching families with young children in their homes, clinicians often find themselves in challenging dual roles. Clinicians intend to be supportive to families by commending strengths and encouraging the bolstering of parenting capacities. However, at the same time, they are also assessing at what point children are unsafe in the care of their families of origin and should instead be in the care of local child welfare authorities. For this reason, the aim of this chapter is to guide clinicians in recognizing parental strengths and capabilities while concurrently assessing for child safety. In making such determinations, however, clinicians may appear to be a threat to parents and, therefore, must also be cognizant of when their own safety could be in jeopardy. Therefore, precautions for clinicians who conduct home assessments are discussed at the end of this chapter.

ASSESSMENT FROM AN ECO-SYSTEMIC PERSPECTIVE

An ecological approach views parents and children not as isolated entities but as part of a complex ecological system. Three major levels of the ecological system are typically identified: the micro-system, mezzo-system, and macro-system (Belsky, 1980; Cicchetti & Lynch, 1993; Mattaini & Meyer, 2002).

The innermost circle is the micro-system, which includes the most immediate entities to the parent and child such as the physical home, relationships between members of the household, and characteristics of the parent and child. The middle circle, the mezzo-system, includes entities in the neighborhood in which the parent and child reside such as social service providers, religious organizations, schools, employers, extended family, and neighbors. The outer circle is the macro-system encompassing the larger societal and cultural attitudes and values affecting parents.

A comprehensive eco-systemic assessment increases the potential for identifying significant protective and risk factors to the parent and child (Oyserman, Mowbray, Allen-Meares, & Firminger, 2000) while enhancing the ability to identify appropriate areas for intervention with families (Hartman, 1995; Mattaini, 1993). The next sections discuss risk and protective factors to be assessed at each of the three main eco-levels.

Micro-system

The home is the center of the family's micro-system. In assessing the physical environment of the home, a primary objective is to identify potential hazards or risks that could seriously compromise a child's physical safety. In addition to the physical appearance of the home, it is important to observe interactions in a natural and familiar setting and to obtain information on familial behavioral patterns (e.g., domestic violence, substance abuse) that can have an impact on a child's well-being.

Home Safety

Several areas of home safety need to be assessed during the home visit. Some may seem obvious to the assessor. However, a parent who was not protected from danger when he or she was a child may not recognize some mundane safety hazards in the home. Sometimes, an unsafe and neglectful environment is readily apparent. One home visited, for instance, was riddled with broken windows; glass shards remained on the floor. Mice were visible. All of the plumbing was in disrepair such that noxious water sat in the sink, the toilet, and the bathtub. It was impossible for the parent or child to bathe or even wash their hands. In other cases, signs of risk are less obvious, so it can be useful to rely on specific assessment criteria.

The following recommendations are adapted from home safety checklists developed by the Illinois Department of Children and Family Services, Office of the Inspector General (1999), based on child injuries investigated in Illinois.

Fires/Burns   To prevent children from suffering burns, homes should have a smoke detector. Matches, lighters, and electrical appliances should be put away where curious children cannot reach them. Some children have suffered serious burns when unmonitored near a stove used to heat the home. Some children who climbed on furniture have been burned after falling and becoming trapped between furniture and a hot radiator. Children have also suffered burns when tap water in the home was erroneously set above 120° F.

Suffocation   It is recommended that parents have cribs for infants. Although it is the norm in some cultures for parents to sleep with their children, occasionally this has resulted in tragedy because a parent rolled over onto his or her child while asleep. Parents who have potential for relapse to substance abuse are at an increased risk for accidental "roll over" death to their infant because these parents are less likely to wake up if they roll onto the child.

Putting children to sleep on their backs significantly reduces the potential for Sudden Infant Death Syndrome (SIDS; National Institute of Child Health and Human Development, n.d.). If a child apparently dies in his sleep, SIDS may be assumed. However, more than one SIDS death in the same family is extremely unlikely and could suggest that one or more children died by deliberate means.

Other areas of safety to assess with regard to risk for suffocation include the accessibility of plastic bags and small toys—equal to or smaller than the diameter of a toilet tissue roll—upon which toddlers might choke. Also, young children can drown in as little as one inch of water, so parents should always monitor children in the bath, near toilets, or when playing near water.

Falls   Infants should not be left on elevated surfaces such as tables, counters, or bunk beds from which they might fall. Beds or furniture a child might climb on should not be placed near windows as some toddlers have found ways to climb out. Parents should also devise barriers to keep children away from stairs.

Poisoning   Parents should put away medications and cleaning fluids so that children do not have access to them. It is important to ask a parent how she administers medication to her child. There have been cases in which a parent, unable to understand prescription directions, overmedicated a child with tragic results. Chipping paint in homes may suggest a potential for lead poisoning to a child eating or breathing in dust. Lead poisoning can result in brain damage to a child. Poisons for rats and mice should not be used or placed where children have access to them. A number of plants are also poisonous (Greene et al., n.d.).

Home Security   It is important to investigate whether a home can be secured. In one case, a parent lived in a home with no locks. Each time the assessor came by there was a different congregation of individuals in the home whom the parent did not know, suggesting that the parent had difficulty establishing protective boundaries for herself and her child.

Family Violence

It is estimated that in 30%–60% of homes where violence exists between partners, child abuse co-occurs (Edleson, 1999). Children can also be harmed by chance while parents are being aggressive to each other or destroying property. Domestic violence can be assessed via several methods. The Conflict Tactics Scale (Straus, 2000) includes questions about the frequency and severity of aggression that partners demonstrate to each other. It can be revealing to ask a parent about the most violent thing he or she has done, or the most violent act his or her partner has perpetrated upon the parent. Inquiry about injuries and/or scars a parent or a child presents with, as well as asking about broken items in the home (e.g., mirrors, lamps, television), can reveal violence in the home. When possible, criminal background checks of all members of the household can be useful. If charges of domestic battery surface, obtaining the police report of particular incidents can be instructive. It is also wise to ask whether firearms are kept in the home. Finally, an assessor can ask children and parents separately about witnessing or participating in physical fighting and aggression in the home, in particular, whether physical fights or aggression have resulted in any injuries and if anyone has ever been hurt to the point of requiring medical care.

Parental Substance Abuse

Substance abuse is a relapsing condition. The more consistent the parent has been in returning to treatment, the greater the chance that he or she may be approaching a more stable period of recovery. As a general rule, about one year of sobriety generally suggests that the parent has developed sufficient coping skills to avoid relapse. It is important to assess whether the parent recognizes that he or she remains vulnerable to relapse and has a prevention plan established, such as calling his or her sponsor, when experiencing increased stress cravings.

While in a home, many valuable clues can be obtained about substance use and abuse. For instance, an assessor can look for signs of substance abuse such as empty alcohol containers, drug paraphernalia, alcohol in the refrigerator, minimal food, or a scarcely furnished home. These may suggest that a parent has spent family income on his or her addiction and/or sold family property to purchase drugs.

Collateral historians can provide invaluable information regarding parental substance use. If the parent is involved in a 12-step program, the sponsor may reveal how well the parent is able to use his or her recovery program to avoid relapse. Other family members or individuals close to the parent can give information about changes in the parent's functioning and use of intoxicating substances. If drug testing has been conducted, reviewing testing results can provide important data.

Parent–Child Interactions

While in the home, an assessor can take advantage of the opportunity to observe spontaneous interactions within the family. In assessing parent–child interaction quality, several aspects warrant close attention (see also Chapter 8).

With young children, it is critical to assess whether the parent is alert to the child's whereabouts. Some parents are so distracted with their own emotional concerns that they may not even hear a child crying and may not be able to adequately monitor a curious toddler (Fraiberg, Adelson, & Shapiro, 1987).

An observer should notice whether a young child uses the parent as a safe base for exploration. Relevant observations include observing how the child orients herself around the parent and whether she leaves the parent to explore her environment but then returns to seek proximity and/or to show the parent what she has found (Bowlby, 1988). When young children do not orient toward parents, it may suggest that the parents have been inconsistent in their responses to their children. Parental inconsistency has been identified as detrimental for child development (Hill & Bush, 2001).

The level of sensitivity that parents demonstrate toward their children and the children's responses to the parents may be indicative of the potential quality of the parent–child relationship as well as level of risk (Crittenden, 1982). High levels of parental insensitivity have been associated with increased risk for abuse, whereas mutually enjoyable interactions between parents and children are a protective factor for abuse (Wolfe, 1991). Parents who are sensitive and able to read children's cues indicative of both physiological and emotional needs are more likely to provide sensitive, safe parenting.

Parents must also be able to assume leadership and caregiving roles with children. Some parents interact with their children more as peers and even invert the parent–child role. Role reversal occurs when parent–child boundaries are blurred. In role-reversed relationships, a child's needs often go unmet while the child is attempting to care for a parent. Role reversal is emotionally burdensome for children as well as developmentally detrimental. One assessment tool that can be helpful in identifying role reversal is the Adult Adolescent Parenting Inventory (Bavolek, 2000).

Evaluators should be alert to signs of hostility or intrusiveness in the parent–child relationship. Does the parent criticize the child or lash out in anger without provocation? Does the parent enter into the child's personal space and ignore the child's cues of discomfort? Does the parent view the child through a negative lens? Negative views of a child have been associated with abuse and negative outcomes for children (Berg-Nielsen, Vikan, & Dahl, 2002). Depressed parents are also more likely to make negative attributions to their child (Azar, Povilaitis, Lauretti, & Pouquette, 1998).

Sometimes parents have unrealistic standards regarding appropriate behavior for young children. When the child fails to meet these standards, the parent attributes negative intent to the child, putting the child at risk for abuse (Azar, Povilaitis et al., 1998). Schmitt (1987) identified seven normal developmental phases as potential triggers for abuse in high-risk families. These "seven deadly sins of childhood" include the following: colic, awakening at night, separation anxiety, normal exploratory behavior, normal negativism, normal to poor appetite, and toilet-training resistance. When a parent expects a young child to be able to sit still, not cry, obey perfectly, and become toilet trained before the child is developmentally capable of these tasks, the parent may feel that the child is purposefully defiant. The resulting parental anger increases the risk for use of overly harsh discipline.

Observing décor in the home can provide additional understanding of the family. Pictures of the children, posted artwork by the children, and availability of toys may indicate some of the value the children have to the parent. It is important to ask about how and where children play. If the family has only a limited number of toys, some parents can be creative in finding ways for children to play with other household items (e.g., pots and pans). On the other hand, a lack of toys could be a result of overly harsh discipline. For example, one parent had thrown out all of her 5-year-old son's toys, including a bicycle, as a consequence for his poor behavior. When energetic children have no place to play and nothing to play with, increased tension and risk can result.

Mezzo-system

The mezzo-system is the second major area of environmental influence. The primary factors affecting parents in their mezzo-system relate to formal and informal social support in the community and the ability to effectively interact on this level of the environment to leverage needed resources.

Social isolation is one of the most clearly identified risk factors for abuse and neglect of children (Gaudin, Polansky, Kilpatrick, & Shilton, 1993; Goldstein, Keller, & Erne, 1985). Belsky (1980) suggested that abuse occurs when stress becomes overwhelming for a parent and intervening social supports are not available to buffer and attenuate emotional response. It has also been suggested that when parents have negative experiences that increase the feelings of vulnerability in other areas of their lives, they may project frustration onto a child and reassert themselves as powerful with abusive acts (Trepper & Barrett, 1989). This idea is consistent with findings that parents who are dissatisfied with their employment have an increased risk for perpetrating child abuse and neglect, and the finding that abuse rates increase in times of high unemployment (Belsky, 1980). Wahler (1980) demonstrated that parents who have fewer and more aversive social contacts also tend to use more coercive parenting tactics. Coercive parenting techniques can have the paradoxical effect of exacerbating the acting-out behaviors that a parent intends to attenuate (Belsky, 1980; Wolfe, 1999). Use of coercion in combination with a child's acting out may then escalate into regular aversive interaction patterns between parents and children, increasing the risk of abuse (Knutson & Bower, 1994). Both harsh discipline and inconsistent discipline have been associated with negative outcomes for children (Berg-Nielsen et al., 2002).

Eco-maps

One tool that can assist assessors in obtaining an initial overview of a parent's interactions in the mezzo-system is an eco-map (Hartman, 1995; Mattaini, 1993). An eco-map is a pictorial representation of a family's interaction with social supports and stressors. To use an eco-map, the assessor sits down with parents at the outset of a home assessment and draws a map of the important people, organizations, and agencies with which the family interacts (e.g., church, employment, social groups, school, legal systems, neighbors, extended family, child care). An eco-map should also indicate the nature of interactions that a parent has identified with various entities (e.g., how positive or negative the interaction is or its level of importance in her life). Eco-maps can illustrate to a parent what areas of support could be further developed to enhance safety for the family (Hartman, 1995). Involving the parent in completing the eco-map can be instructive and empowering for the parent (Kemp, Whittaker, & Tracy, 1997). Additional eco-maps can be completed over time to illustrate progress and to assist in setting future goals for developing social support (Mattaini, 1993).

Given the now well-established association between child abuse and neglect with social isolation (Belsky, 1980; Gaudin et al., 1993; Polansky, 1986; Polansky, Gaudin, Ammon, & Davis, 1985), the eco-map is particularly appropriate when issues of child safety are to be assessed.

Assessing Social Supports

When interviewing parents about social supports, it is important to keep in mind that sometimes parents have more social support than they give themselves credit for. A depressed mood may contribute to a parent having a more negative view of the willingness of people around her to help. Probing about whom a parent has sought out or might seek out in the future in particular situations can bring up a number of supportive individuals. Specific to parenting, the Arizona Social Support Inventory (Barrera, 1981) includes questions such as who a parent would go to if she wanted advice in handling her child's behavior, who could lend her $25 if she needed it for something important for her child, and who could care for her child if the parent had to be hospitalized. After completing the questionnaire, assessors can follow up with the identified supports to determine whether they are available for the parent in the future.

Critical Assessment of Informal Social Supports   Parents with serious mental illness and parents with a history of abuse and/or neglect may have difficulty in both establishing and maintaining supportive relationships with friends and relatives (Crittenden, 1996; Mowbray, Oyserman, Zemencuk, & Ross, 1995). In some cases, the parent's identified support system may not be helpful in enhancing safety, but instead increases the risk for the parent and her child. Some parents identify individuals with whom they use drugs or alcohol as their support system. Others identify abusive and transient partners (Mowbray et al., 1995).

Sometimes in severely impoverished neglectful families, familial support has little to offer the parent and child. The parent offers little stimulation to the child, and relatives may reinforce the parent's limited involvement and attention to the child (Crittenden, 1996). In such families, all members may have a sense of powerlessness of themselves and others that is associated with lethargy and depression (Crittenden, 1996).

Neglect has been argued to be the most damaging form of child maltreatment. (Egeland & Erickson, 1987; Shakel, 1987). One parent, her mother, and her brother reported that they all assisted each other in caring for the parent's infant; nevertheless, the child was diagnosed with nonorganic failure to thrive. Outside of her family setting—in the hospital and then in a foster home—the child responded eagerly to caregiving and easily gained weight. The parent and her family had been unable to recognize and provide for the infant's emotional and physiological needs.

Assessing Formal Sources of Support   Lack of high-quality services for parents with serious mental illness is generally accepted (Nicholson & Biebel, 2002; Ramchandani & Stein, 2003). As such, and given possibly limited economic means, assessing the ability of parents to leverage the limited resources available to them becomes important. Some important neighborhood resources include public transportation, grocery stores, potential employers, hospitals, mental health care providers, substance abuse treatment, 12-step groups, food pantries, schools, and social services agencies. Some services that have been specifically shown to decrease the risk of child abuse and neglect include child respite centers and home visiting programs (Daro, 1996). With an eye to child development, sites for potential positive shared experiences for parents and children such as public libraries, public parks, swimming pools, boys and girls clubs, and adult supervised extracurricular activities for older children are important resources.

The number of services immediately available in any one community is less important than the parent's ability to procure what she needs from her environment. Part of assessing a parent's resourcefulness is determining how aware she is of services around her, whether she seeks out services when needed, and whether she can also accept assistance when offered. When a parent is less aware of services available to her, she can be offered referrals, but at times, merely offering an agency name and phone number will not result in the parent receiving the needed help (Kemp et al., 1997).

In some cases, depressive symptoms (e.g., depressed mood, lack of will, lethargy, inability to concentrate, decreased interest in pleasurable activities) interfere with a parent's energy level and motivation to seek out services or even consider that there might be help available for the family. Other times, cognitive limitations, an inability to read, or language difficulties inhibit a parent's ability to secure what she needs from her environment. In such situations, the assessor can make efforts to remove barriers for the parent. In the case of a depressed, socially isolated parent, an assessor can first be hopeful for the client that things can get better (Walsh, 1999). The assessor can temporarily escort a parent to appointments, demonstrating how to take public transportation to important locales. The assessor making phone calls with a parent to seek out important services models important resource leveraging skills. The assessor's persistent involvement can also show the parent how to be tenacious in following up when a needed resource is not immediately forthcoming. A parent may need reminder calls (or visits) about appointments and even about taking medications for a while. As the parent's depression improves, the assessor is likely to see the parent becoming more capable of being independently resourceful, no longer requiring the same level of hands-on assistance.

One aspect of being resourceful is having an ability to trust that some people can be helpful and that things occasionally may go well. Having an amiable nature and the ability to develop and maintain relationships with service providers—assessors like to be of assistance and go to extra effort—is a boon. Some parents have maintained long-term relationships with mental health service coordinators or former child welfare service coordinators who report they will always make themselves available to the particular client to help him or her seek out resources as needs arise.

Other parents, unfortunately, have had such negative and traumatic experiences with social-service providers that they have a generalized belief that everyone is out to get them, and they resist attempts others make to help. They may sabotage services and resources with their attitude. Sometimes, this distrust rises to the level of a delusion, a fixed false belief. Delusions are treatment resistant; this psychotic symptom is infrequently attenuated by psychotropic medications. People experiencing paranoid delusions will seldom take medications, believing that the person offering the medication is attempting to poison them. If the parent does not take advantage of services suggested despite honest efforts of mental health workers to identify and remove barriers, she is less likely to be able to secure services in the near future, and her child's needs may go unmet.

Involvement in Religious Institutions or Other Social Organizations   Parents who have extensive extrafamilial support are often involved in religious communities. Although some religious communities do not support the use of psychotropic medications, a perspective which would be detrimental to seriously mentally ill parents, many religious communities provide tremendous benefits to families. ByBee, Mowbray, Oyserman, and Lewandowski (2003) found that parents who perceived themselves as religious and regularly attended church services had higher levels of community functioning than parents who did not. Participation in a faith community often gives a parent a sense of belonging and meaning. Peers within a faith community can provide a vast array of assistance to parents. One parent who was an active member in a Jehovah's Witness Kingdom Hall was able to identify mentors for each of her five children in foster care. When the mentors were contacted, each reported having known the parent for many years and were familiar with the children's significant behavioral problems. Mentors reported that they met with the child they mentored weekly for Bible study. Should the children return home, the mentors were prepared to assist with transportation, monitoring of the children after school, and academic tutoring. Mentors were also prepared to occasionally allow the children to stay at their houses overnight to give the parent respite. The involvement of the mother in this community and her willingness to ask for and receive specific assistance for her children vastly improved her potential to resume the role of primary caregiver for her children.

Another important extrafamilial support system can be 12-step groups such as Narcotics Anonymous or Alcoholics Anonymous. Not all parents find these groups helpful, but some are able to rely on them for broad peer support in maintaining sobriety. One parent living near the residential treatment center from which she graduated networked with other graduates from the same program who had been successful in having children returned to them from Child Protective Services. These women assisted each other with transportation, child care, emotional support, and stress management.

Family History   A critical factor that influences a mother's ability to establish and maintain supports both in her family and in the larger community and environment is her own family history and structure. Diagramming this structure in the form of a genogram can provide an understanding of historical patterns in a parent's family of origin and her current family system (Hartman, 1995; McGoldrick, Gerson, & Shellenberger, 1999). Three to four generations are typically included in a genogram, which provides a visual overview of a family's history and structure, including relevant marriages and relationships, children, deaths, and births. Because support systems are so crucial for parents with mental illness, it is useful to include in the genogram people who have played important ongoing roles in the parent and child's lives, such as foster parents and stepparents. Together, the assessor and the parent can generate hypotheses regarding familial caregiving patterns. Such understanding may provide guidance for a parent in decision making for her family's future.

Extended family members' understanding of and attitudes toward mental illness can affect a parent's acceptance of her mental illness and the parent's potential for maintaining treatment compliance. When family members are supportive of a parent in maintaining her health and participating in treatment, the parent is more likely to develop a pattern of consistent medication and psychosocial treatment compliance over time (Battaglia, 2001). Family members can also have the opposite affect, however. Family members may discourage medication use. One family insisted that a parent who was being assessed was not ill but was using her diagnosed mental illness as an excuse to be lazy. The family regularly dissuaded the parent from taking medication; family members did not realize that they were further debilitating the parent.

Some families recognize the presence of an illness, yet avoid the relative with mental illness because the family is unsure of how to interact with anyone who suffers from mental illness. Sometimes when family issues such as these emerge, a family conference can be called so that service providers may share information about mental illness and catalyze discussion regarding how family members can be supportive. It can also be the case, however, that the parent ostracizes herself from her family secondary to paranoia or other behavior associated with psychosis.

It is well established that a history of physical abuse or neglect in a family increases risk for repeating problematic familial patterns with one's own children (Belsky, 1980; Crittenden, 1996). Individuals having a history of physical abuse are more likely to hold attitudes accepting potentially injurious punitive discipline as normative (e.g., hitting with an object). People with a history of physical abuse are also more likely to use physical punishment and have a lower tolerance for irritating child behaviors such that they are at greater risk for disciplinary escalation (Knutson & Bower, 1994). A history of abuse and neglect does not predetermine a parent to become abusive and neglectful to his or her child, however.

One known mediating factor associated with whether a parent repeats or does not repeat patterns of abuse with her children is the parent's current state of mind regarding childhood caregivers who may have perpetrated abuse or neglect to her. As noted in Chapter 5, one way to assess this is to use the AAI (Hesse, 1999). The main point of this interview is to determine if parents have been able to develop integrated and coherent understandings of experiences with their own childhood caregivers that would allow them to alter problematic familial behavioral patterns.

When a parent can speak about childhood loss and trauma in a coherent manner, setting former caregivers in a relevant context and criticizing them with a sense of proportion, balance, and even humor, the parent is more likely to be capable of providing emotionally sensitive and secure care to her child. In contrast, parents are more likely to unwittingly repeat past problematic familial caregiving patterns and have difficulty providing emotional sensitivity and security to a child if they speak of their developmental history in a more confusing and less consistent manner. For example, some parents give overly positive reports of caregivers but are unable to back up these reports with relevant examples, and/or they give incongruent examples of caregivers having been abusive and neglectful. Other parents minimize the importance of relationships with their caregivers, for example, admitting to having suffered neglect or abuse but suggesting that it was not at all painful or meaningful to the parent. Then again, other parents become disorganized and preoccupied when discussing their history of loss and/or abuse. Parents may give overly lengthy reports; appear angry, passive, fearful; or give seemingly illogical responses such as speaking of someone who has died as if he or she was still alive. In these instances, a parent may be at a greater risk for unwittingly repeating problematic familial behavioral patterns (Hesse, 1999).

Macro-system

One of the most significant macro-systemic issues affecting quality of parenting is poverty, unemployment, and the stress associated with poor economic conditions (Belsky, 1980; Blanch et al., 1994; Gaudin et al., 1993; Gil, 1987). Child neglect is associated with poverty. At-risk parents and children, including parents with serious mental illness, are often dependent on limited public resources for economic support (Azar et al., 1998; Crittenden, 1996; Mowbray et al., 1995). It follows that the stress a parent experiences in an economic context may exacerbate the stress she experiences in interactions with her child. Belsky (1980) documented the positive correlation of unemployment and child abuse rates.

A lack of stable and safe housing is associated with poverty. Stable, safe housing for a person with limited resources is also a major issue for parents who are seriously mentally ill. Assessors must distinguish between housing issues that are a result of a housing shortage versus a parent being unable to maintain housing because of her illness. Although affordable and safe low-income housing in the United States is not abundant, it is not impossible for a parent with serious mental illness to secure adequate housing for her family. In some cases, parents have familial support such that the parent and her children may live in the same household with mentally healthy relatives. Sometimes, a family member who owns housing rents a unit to a parent with mental illness at a reduced rate, or relatives assist in subsidizing rent. Such arrangements require the parent to be capable of maintaining positive relationships with family members.

Sometimes parents have worked with service providers for access to public housing programs or rare residential programs designed especially for parents with severe mental illness (Cohler, Stott, & Musick, 1996). In certain cases, however, a parent will unlikely remain in stable housing. Many parents who have family members willing to assist them experience paranoia such that they are always concerned about the motives of family members and, therefore, avoid the assistance family members or others proffer. Utilization of family funds for substance use may compromise a parent's ability to maintain housing. Parents with personality disorders may have difficulty maintaining housing more for emotional reasons than for issues of the housing supply. One parent, secondary to repeated severe trauma (e.g., witnessing a parent's murder, suffering repeated sexual abuse, having a child murdered by a family member), had been running away from homes from the time she was 5 years old. She had been unable to remain in one location for more than a few months throughout latency, adolescence, and early adulthood. Despite the fact that she loved her son, had regular contact with him, and interacted well with him, she could not provide him with the stable environment he required.

Another important macro-level issue is that of culture, values, and community norms with respect to violence. Belsky (1980) argued the American culture tolerates an unconscionable level of violence, pointing out that the United States has much higher rates of violent crime than other developed countries. Families who live in areas in which violence is common may have regularly witnessed acts of violence such that they develop a greater acceptance of aggressive coping strategies. In the late 1980s on the south side of Chicago, for instance, 40% of teenagers reported having witnessed a shooting, one fourth had seen someone killed, and one fourth had been a victim of violence (e.g., shot or stabbed; Jenkins & Bell, 1997). Coming from a community of heightened violence may decrease the threshold for people within that area to use aggression.

Assessors must take community context into consideration when evaluating parents. The community from which a parent comes is particularly important with respect to deciding if reported behaviors can be considered deviant and diagnosable (American Psychiatric Association, 2000). For example, if a parent had gang involvement during adolescence such that she was involved in violent activities, a clinician from another socioeconomic background might consider diagnosing antisocial personality traits. If nearly all teenagers growing up in that area, however, were involved with gangs, it would be more difficult to support such a diagnosis. Bestowing such a diagnosis, despite the parent's context, may unjustly bias the child welfare system against the parent. Critical information would need to be gathered from people who knew the parent as an adolescent to determine if the parent was more violent than other youth in her neighborhood or if she was quite similar to others using gang membership as a survival strategy in a tough area.

It is also important to consider how racial, ethnic, and community culture affects parents' views of themselves in the community. People of color can and do experience stress due to prejudice. Learning how a parent perceives her own culture and the culture at large is, therefore, critical (Castillo, 1997). A good time to ask about culture is while completing a family genogram. It is important to know whether a client felt that he or she or his or her family was much different from other families in the area in which he or she was raised. For example, if a mother has a child at a young age, it is important to know how she views this. Is she following cultural and familial patterns of generally having children at a young age, or does she feel that she has failed in some way because she had a child when she was too young?

Religious beliefs are also often culturally bound and contribute to a parent's view of herself in the world. These can be identified as protective or risk factors depending on how they have served the parent. A faithful parent can maintain hope in dire circumstances (Walsh, 1999). Sometimes we need to ask others from the parent's community about how a community operates in order to distinguish whether certain descriptions a parent provides are cultural or psychotic (American Psychiatric Association, 2000). For example, one client repeatedly reported that God spoke to her. When her pastor was consulted by the social worker, he explained that in their Pentecostal faith it was common in the congregation for members to say that God spoke to them.

When a parent is an immigrant or her family has recently immigrated, assessors can ask where the parent's family is from and pose questions about the family's immigration history. When a parent speaks another language, it is optimal to refer the client to a mental health worker who speaks the parent's language. When this is not possible, a translator is required. Optimally, translators should be professionally trained and certified in translation to decrease bias and miscommunication. Translators may be able to explain cultural attitudes related to mental illness, child rearing, and involvement with authoritative figures.

Empirical studies suggest that sexual orientation of a caregiver alone does not jeopardize the general well-being of children (American Psychological Association, 2001). A parent may, nevertheless, be affected by stigma and prejudice complicating child custody issues. A good way to ask about sexual identity that demonstrates an acceptance of the client regardless of sexual orientation is to ask whether a parent has had male and female sexual partners and relationships and to which gender the parent is attracted. In one assessment, it was necessary to advocate for a mother who possessed adequate parenting skills but who had been in same-sex relationships. A significant amount of bias developed around this particular issue, delaying the return of her child.

SAFETY ISSUES FOR ASSESSORS

The home visit is an essential part of a comprehensive assessment of parenting competency and risk (Budd & Holdsworth, 1996); therefore, it should not be forfeited in most situations. Home visits provide rich, naturalistic information on family functioning and safety. Visiting the home can also help an evaluator confirm or qualify observations made in other settings. It is useful for assessors to be sensitive to the meaning clients attribute to a home visit. Some clients develop a stronger rapport with assessors because the assessor made extra effort to see the client's surroundings, and the home visit may have decreased the client's burden of travel to an office visit. Other clients, however, feel intruded upon.

It is important that assessors take necessary precautions to ensure their own safety. It should be routine for assessors to carry a cellular phone and ensure that co-workers are aware of where and when home visits are being conducted. Some service providers only send out home visitors in pairs. When the community in which the parent lives is violent, the parent herself or others in the community may steer assessors toward safer times to visit. In one Chicago community, a gang war was taking place, but community members recommended assessors visit the parent in the mornings as all shootings occurred after schools let out for the day at 2:30 p.m.

Sometimes, the parent, herself, poses risk to the assessor. To minimize such risk, having a first meeting with any parent in an office setting can be advantageous so that rapport can be established before the home visit. It is useful to review available records before visiting the home to determine whether a client has a known history of violence, has impulse control difficulties, or has previously been threatening to other mental health workers. When a parent has been violent to other mental health workers, obviating the home visit may be best, and extra security may even be needed in the office setting, particularly when assessors have to present potentially upsetting information. It can be useful to develop relationships with local police who can be available in the rare circumstances in which there is a risk of aggression. Also rare, but possible, is parents becoming focused on a particular assessor either as a target for anger or as a focus of delusional romantic involvement. All assessors should take the general precautions of maintaining an unlisted phone number and a mailing address separate from their residence to make it more difficult for an angry or infatuated client to contact an assessor at home.

CONCLUSION

The ability of a parent with serious mental illness to maintain a safe home environment, to request and accept assistance from informal and formal social supports around him or her, and to manage societal pressures associated with prejudice and oppression can significantly enhance or diminish his or her overall ability to provide care to his or her child(ren). As such, a comprehensive eco-systemic environmental assessment of the parent is essential. Assessment requires mental health professionals to recognize both risk and protective factors with which parents present. Child safety is paramount. Parents with histories of having been victims of abuse can provide critical information about the degree to which past problematic familial patterns may be repeated unwittingly in the future. Having an integrated understanding of traumatic experiences from childhood decreases the chance of continuing a cycle of abuse, whereas a less coherent understanding of these experiences is less auspicious. Although assessors are determining the degree of safety in the homes of families, they must also be cognizant of and take proactive steps to protect themselves.

8

Children's Perspectives and Needs

Lucia was 10 years old when her mother tried to overdose on medication. The overdose occurred in the context of Mrs. Adams' depression, which had been triggered by the death of her husband earlier that year. When Mrs. Adams slipped into her bedroom one morning and locked the door, Lucia suspected that her mother was thinking of committing suicide. Lucia knocked repeatedly on the door, pleading with her to stop. When her mother did not answer, Lucia became desperate and called relatives for help. Even after her mother's illness symptoms had remitted, Lucia remained anxious about her mother's well-being. She monitored her mother's whereabouts constantly and grew both angry and anxious when she could not locate her.

As the above vignette illustrates, children are deeply affected by mental illness in a parent. However, not all children are equally overt in showing how maternal mental illness affects them. Some children function well and are resilient by all outward appearances (Rutter, 1985). At the same time, resilience often comes at a high cost to children. Although they can cope well and show high levels of achievement, resilient children may experience underlying feelings of loss, responsibility, guilt, and anguish (Marsh, 1998).

Regardless of how readily children express concerns and vulnerability, most are affected to some degree by mental illness in a parent (Beardslee et al., 1998; Rutter, 1986). Some children worry about their parent's well-being. Others become pulled into their parent's psychiatric symptoms and may come to see the world in a depressive, obsessive, or psychotic way. Yet, others assume the role of a parent or worry that they, themselves, will become mentally ill or develop similar kinds of symptoms.

Children of parents with diagnosable mental disorders are vulnerable in other ways, too. Studies estimate that about one third to one half of children whose parents have major mental illness will develop a psychiatric illness themselves (Hammen & Brennan, 2003; Rutter, 1986), twice the amount of children born to parents without major mental illness. They are also more likely than other children to have insecure attachment patterns with their caregivers (Hipwell, Goossens, Melhuish, & Kumar, 2000) and experience interpersonal and behavioral difficulties (Beardslee et al., 1998). Exposure to a parent's psychiatric symptoms appears to be especially detrimental if experienced in the early years of development when a child is still dependent on the parent for survival (Lyons-Ruth, Wolfe, & Lyubchik, 2000; Murray et al., 1999).

This chapter focuses on children's perspectives and needs. It presents an overview about how parental mental illness can affect children's well-being and development, followed by an overview of the child assessment.

HOW PARENTAL MENTAL ILLNESS AFFECTS CHILDREN

Parental mental illness can affect children's well-being and development in different ways. Risk may be transmitted genetically to a child. Direct exposure to the parent's illness or indirect exposure via poor parenting or marital discord can also have an impact on children. The effect on children's development may occur through factors associated with mental illness such as poverty, social adversity, and disadvantage. Genetic factors can also interact with environmental factors to affect child outcome.

Parental mental illness does not affect children equally. A child with a difficult temperament, for instance, may elicit different responses from a parent than a child with an easy temperament, thereby contributing to a more difficult parenting pathway and to a less favorable outcome for the child.

According to the stress-diathesis theory (Goodman & Gotlib, 1999), genetic and early environmental factors interact with later environmental stresses to precipitate the onset of a psychiatric disorder in a child or trigger a relapse of illness symptoms (Sullivan, Neale, & Kendler, 2000). A child whose mother experiences serious anxiety symptoms when the child is young, for instance, may be genetically more vulnerable to developing panic attacks, but she may only experience such symptoms in later childhood or adolescence, when she is under high levels of stress.

Poor mental health and developmental outcomes are more likely if children experience multiple risk factors, including both parents with mental illness, poor parenting, marital discord, or maltreatment (Goodman & Gotlib, 1999). Poor outcomes have also been associated with how severe the parent's illness is (Foley et al., 2001). Having a secure attachment to the mother or to other family members can lower the risk, as can a positive sense of self and good coping skills (Goodman & Gotlib, 1999). Outcomes in children are also likely to be more positive if the mother's illness is relatively mild and not chronic (Radke-Yarrow, McCann, DeMulder, Belmont, Martinez, & Richardson, 1995).

CHILDREN'S RESPONSES TO MENTAL ILLNESS IN A PARENT

Children respond in different ways to mental illness in a parent. Some children assume a parental role so as to fill gaps in family functioning. Others may blame themselves for their parent's illness or may become self-sufficient, feeling that they can do without a parent or support. The next section considers a variety of responses that are often observed in children of parents with mental illness.

Am I to Blame?

Feeling that they are to blame is a common struggle for many children who have a mother with a psychiatric disorder. Children will try, in their own way, to make sense of their mother's behavior. If they find that their mother is irritable, depressed, angry, or psychotic, children may conclude that they caused their mother's depression or psychosis, or they may feel that they caused their mother to feel irritable, depressed, or angry or to become psychotic. Unless corrected, these feelings of responsibility for a parent's illness are likely to persist over time and will contribute to a child feeling that he or she is constantly to blame for what happens.

Communications from parents or other adults in the family can exacerbate this situation (Bowlby, 1988). The following types of communications, for instance, are especially likely to increase a child's sense of blame: telling a child that her behavior is making the parent ill, blaming the child directly for the illness, or telling the child that her behavior is driving the parent "crazy."

Due to their dependence on their parents for love and survival, young children readily believe what their parents tell them and are likely to conclude that their behavior has contributed to their parent's symptoms. Some children may express their feelings of guilt openly. Others, as you will see in the next vignette, express their guilt through their behavior.

Lillian, age 4 years, was seen in a clinic after her mother had been hospitalized for symptoms associated with bipolar disorder. Lillian's father was concerned because Lillian scratched her arms until they bled. She also pinched her cheeks repeatedly. It soon became clear that Lillian was inflicting the wounds as a way of blaming herself for her mother's illness. Her feelings of blame had been fueled by an aunt's statement that Lillian's "bad" behavior was making her mother ill.

Intensified Self-Sufficiency

Some children become precociously self-sufficient in response to mental illness in a parent. A child who does this adapts her behavior to make things work within a family that is under considerable strain (Lieberman, 1993). In essence, a child with intensified self-sufficiency tries hard to fill in the gaps in family functioning by compensating for a parent who is absent to some degree. Some children, as Henry in the next vignette, take on the role of parent early on.

Just prior to his birth, Henry's mother had been diagnosed with schizoaffective disorder, a chronic disorder that includes mood swings and psychotic episodes. Although he was only 4 years old, Henry was highly self-sufficient. He packed his own lunches for preschool and walked down the street alone to purchase milk and bread for his mother.

Intensified self-sufficiency often builds on a child's need to control situations to obtain some outward security about what he can expect (Lieberman, 1993). Although sometimes viewed as mature, extreme self-sufficiency comes at a high emotional cost to a child (Bowlby, 1988). Children who are highly self-sufficient, for instance, have great difficulties in relying on adults for any help or support, insisting instead that they can do it by themselves.

Role Reversal

Role reversal refers to a child feeling compelled to enact or fill a parental role (Byng-Hall, 2002). As a defense, it shares similarities to self-sufficiency in that it builds on a child's need to control situations to obtain some sense of outward security. Although more common in older children (Jurkovic, 1997), even very young children may reverse roles and act like a parent to fill gaps in family functioning (Boris, Wheeler, Heller, & Zeanah, 2000). Children who evidence role reversal often hope that they can change a parent's psychiatric symptoms and that a real relationship with the parent will be possible if they could only care enough for her (Winnicott, 1965).

Some argue that role reversal is adaptive since a child learns responsibility and useful organizational skills at an early age (Göpfert, Webster, & Nelki, 2004a). Role reversal does become a concern if the child misses out on being a child, if too heavy of responsibilities are placed on the child's shoulders, or if it constricts the child's own development and his or her capacities to feel and learn.

Key questions that can help a clinician to determine whether role reversal is becoming too much for a child include the following: To what extent is the child assuming an adult role in the family? How long has the child been assuming this role? Is the child's need to fill an adult role seriously compromising the child's emotional well-being and her zest for learning and exploration?

Loneliness, Embarrassment, and Confusion

Marsh (1998) referred to the impact of parental mental illness on family members as a "burden." For children, part of this burden includes grieving for a parent they knew and loved before the illness set in. Another part of the burden is that children are often confronted with the objective burden of coping with caregiving responsibilities, the parent's symptoms, and the social stigma of the illness.

Both burdens are stressful for children. As a result, many children who have a parent with a chronic mental illness experience a profound sense of loneliness or confusion about their lives at home. Children may wonder, for instance, whether they are the only one who has a mother with serious mental problems, or whether others will believe what they say. Some children may feel they have no one to talk with about their experiences at home. Others may feel confused about their mother's symptoms or lack a sense of what is normal behavior or routine in families. For some children, it is hard to decipher which experiences are normal and which are not (Marsh, 1998).

Some children feel guilty that they were spared the illness and are healthy. Others may experience embarrassment by their mothers' symptoms or at odd mannerisms or behaviors they might engage in. One child felt embarrassed because her mother acted in a strange way when others came to visit the home. Another child worried that her mother would come to school when she was depressed or manic. The child also felt she couldn't bring friends home because the house was always messy.

Compensation, Distortion, and Secrecy

Many families hide the fact that a parent or other family member has a mental illness or substance abuse problem (Kroll, 2004; Ostler et al., 2007). Some families are silent and do not discuss the illness. Others fail to acknowledge it openly outside the family. Yet, in other families the illness may be acknowledged, but symptoms may be minimized, distorted, or changed in ways that are confusing to children.

The stigma of mental illness, misunderstandings about the illness and its nature, loyalty to the family, and fear of experiencing adverse reactions from others are key factors that contribute to secrecy or distorted communication patterns in families (Fitzpatrick, Reder, & Lucey, 1995). If a child is in foster care, the need to keep family problems secret may be intensified even more, especially if the child feels that revealing family problems may lead to a long-term or even permanent separation from the parent.

Secretive and distorted family communication patterns make it difficult for children to obtain an objective context and conceptual framework for understanding the effects of the mental illness on the family, on themselves, and on relationships. Such communication patterns, coupled with the belief that expressing one's own needs would be too much for the family to handle, can also contribute to a child needing to hide his or her own feelings and needs from others (Bowlby, 1988).

In extreme cases, children who deny or suppress their own feelings and thoughts develop a false sense of self (Miller, 1983). Children with a false sense of self essentially deny their own feelings or thoughts and try to do or be what they think is "right" for others in the family. Some children in this situation try to be perfect or reach an ideal for which the parent wishes. Underlying the child's outward appearance of perfection, however, is the fundamental fear that she is not good enough (Lieberman, 1993). By trying to be perfect, the child may unconsciously believe that the parent will become better or that the parent may be more able or willing to respond to the child's needs.

Involvement in a Parent's Symptoms

Children who live alone with a mother who has a psychiatric disorder and who are the focus of the mother's own unresolved needs or conflicts may become entangled in their mother's illness to the detriment of their own development.

Entanglement in a mother's psychiatric symptoms may take different forms. If the mother is seriously depressed, highly anxious, or obsessive, a child may come to see the world in a more negative, anxious, or compulsive way than is warranted. Some children become entangled in the illness by becoming the mother's confidant and by sharing her secrets and fears. Children who live in these circumstances may be burdened with and ultimately overwhelmed with too much information. Rather than calming the child, the mother's difficulties in containing her own worries may leave the child with often unbearable levels of anxiety (Symington & Symington, 1999).

Some children closely identify with a mother with mental illness and may interpret their own behavior as early symptoms of their mother's disorder. Children in this situation tend to keep these worries to themselves. Only when they trust a person well do they even begin to reveal that they fear they are developing symptoms similar to their parents'. Worries about becoming like the mother who is ill are more likely if family members worry about the child or note that she is like the parent who is ill (Hall, 2004).

Other children may enter into their mothers' psychotic worlds by accepting their mothers' psychotic beliefs as their own. This situation tends to occur in children and parents who are socially isolated. It may be a way for the child to feel close to a parent who is hard to reach emotionally. The following is an example of a *folie à deux*—a situation in which the child shares the parent's delusional state (Anthony, 1971):

Rachel, age 12, had been raised alone by her mother since birth. The two had little contact with other family members due largely to her mother's delusional disorder. Because she was socially isolated, Rachel listened constantly to her mother. Over time, she came to accept many of her mother's delusions as true. She fully believed, for instance, that others outside of the family were trying to poison them.

Separations and Foster Care

Clinical studies estimate as many as 60%–80% of parents with major mental illness may lose or relinquish custody of their children in their lives, either temporarily or permanently (Coverdale & Aruffo, 1989; Nicholson et al., 2001). As a result, children born to a mother with major mental illness are prone to experience frequent disruptions in care (Caton et al., 1998). If a parent is hospitalized for a period of time or experiences severe illness exacerbations, the child may stay with the non–mentally ill parent or with relatives or friends until the parent stabilizes and recovers. Others may be placed in foster care until a decision about custody is made (Gruenbaum & Gammeltoft, 1993; Ruppert & Bagedahl-Strindlund, 2001).

If the mother is absent, either physically or psychologically, the child is likely to experience not only the loss of a healthy mother and loss of a normal family life but also a loss of stability and confidence. Some children feel that they lose a sense of who they are and what they want for themselves in life. In essence, children growing up in these circumstances are at risk for losing sight of their own needs and of the ability to control their lives (Marsh,1998).

Some children who experience prolonged separations from a mother with a mental illness maintain a secret relationship with her in their minds. They may dream about the parent, wait for letters, and fantasize that she will return to or be available for them. Children who maintain a relationship with a "hidden parent" idealize the relationship and continue to organize their feelings and behaviors around the absent parent (Jolowicz, 1969).

Helping a child who idealizes a parent to recognize the painful reality of separation and loss is an essential part of the therapeutic work that is needed to help the child onto a healthier pathway. As necessary and important as this is, it can be an arduous task for children to put the pieces together and understand that their parents have been absent from their lives.

THE CHILD ASSESSMENT

A grounded understanding of how mental illness in a parent can affect a child's development, attachment bond, mental health, and well-being provides the conceptual basis for the child assessment. Overarching goals of the child assessment are to establish what a child's needs are, identify interventions that could help the child onto a healthier pathway, and determine the fit between a child's needs and a parent's caregiving skills (Reder & Lucey, 1995b).

In the child assessment, the clinician determines what the child's attachment relationship is to the parent and what the child's perspective is on the parent–child relationship. It is important to understand whether the child has become negatively involved in the mother's psychiatric symptoms, what his or her current functioning is in relevant areas of development, whether he or she has special medical, psychological, or other needs, and what the child's relationships are with others within and outside of the family (Göpfert et al., 2004a; Jacobsen et al., 1997; Reder & Lucey, 1995b).

Two or more sessions (1–2 hours each) are usually needed to complete the child assessment. The clinician's role is to engage the child in the assessment and to find out what the child's perspectives, feelings, and needs are without taxing the child to go beyond his or her attention span, ability, and interest. As part of the assessment process, the clinician pays close attention to the way the child talks about the parent, how he or she copes under stress, what his or her strengths are, and how he or she relates to the clinician and others.

When the child assessment is completed, the clinician will have information on the following areas:

- The child's attachment quality (relationship) to the parent

- How the child relates to and maintains relationships with others

- What the child's coping skills and strengths are

- What the child's sense of self is like

- How the child regulates affect, especially anger, fear, and pain

- Whether the child has special needs and what these consist of

Sources of Information

A good place to start with an inquiry into a child's needs is to obtain all relevant records on the child, including child welfare records, medical records, school records, and any existing psychological or psychiatric records. A thorough record review is supplemented with an interview and observations of the child. In addition, the clinician will screen for mental health problems and for delays in development. Interviewing adults who know the child well (e.g., parent, foster parents, teachers, mental health professionals) complements these data, providing additional perspectives on and information about a child's current needs and developmental trajectory. Such interviews will inquire into diverse areas of functioning, including medical, educational, psychiatric, emotional, and developmental issues.

An assessment of the child should be closely guided by what is developmentally relevant to the child's current stage. It will also be tailored to address the specific issues raised by the child and her unique experiences within the family. Children who have experienced maternal depression, for instance, may evidence delays in their cognitive, emotional, and behavioral functioning (Murray et al., 1999). Given these associations, assessors will select screening tools that can identify children's level of functioning in these specific areas of development.

The aim of the child assessment is to obtain enough information to understand what the critical experiences are that have helped to define who this child is and how she is functioning emotionally and developmentally. Focusing on who the child has had close relationships with, how these adults have responded to the child, and how the child feels about such relationships and their importance in her life are essential to help a clinician to define family and relationship factors that have contributed to a child's sense of self and well-being. As experiences in the child's life are sorted through, the clinician draws conclusions about the child's attachment quality, her responses to the parent's mental illness, as well as the child's unique needs and strengths. Each of these areas is discussed in more detail in the next sections.

The Parent–Child Attachment Relationship

Understanding the nature and quality of the parent–child attachment relationship is the centerpiece of the child assessment. An attachment figure is the person the child seeks out under stress (Ainsworth, Blehar, Waters, & Wall, 1978). It is the person the child prefers over others when consolation, help, or support are needed. Usually, it is the person who can best comfort and advise the child. A child typically forms a primary attachment to the person who takes care of the child and responds to her on a daily basis (Bowlby, 1988). Typically, this person is the child's parent.

The presence or absence of the attachment figure, and the quality of the relationship between that person and the child influence every aspect of a child's development (Bowlby, 1988; Lieberman, 1993). Children derive their sense of worth from how they are seen in the eyes of the parent (Bowlby, 1988). Children also learn from their attachment figure how to know when it is safe to explore on their own and when it is dangerous. In this way, a child comes to develop a sense of inner trust in the possibility of feeling secure and protected, while learning to become independent (Lieberman, 1993).

Because a child's early attachment relationships become a template for how the child forms later relationships in life, assessing such relationships can help clinicians to understand whether the child is self-reliant or fragile, whether the child feels alone or endangered, and whether the child sees the world as a reason for concern or as a source of security and support (Lieberman, 1993).

Attachment behavior is most obvious when a child is frightened, fatigued, sick, alone, or in an unknown environment (Bowlby, 1988). Observing interactions between a parent and child under stress, then, can provide telling clues as to the quality and nature of an attachment relationship (Ainsworth et al., 1978). A child who seeks out the parent directly for comfort or asks for help feels more security in his or her relationship to the parent than a child who is unable to turn to the parent and denies that he or she needs any help or a child who becomes scattered or falls apart emotionally under stress.

Attachment Measures

The standard attachment observation that is often used in research to identify parent–child attachment quality in infancy and early childhood is the Strange Situation (Ainsworth et al., 1978). This observation consists of several carefully timed episodes designed to activate a young child's attachment system due to a combination of a new situation, a stranger, and brief separations from the parent (or caregiver). Based on the child's behavior toward the parent upon two reunions, one of four attachment patterns is identified in infants and young children (Solomon & George, 1999).

In the secure attachment pattern, a child is able to use the parent as a secure base. He or she directly seeks out the parent for comfort under stress. Once comforted, the child is then able to return to exploring the world. In this pattern, there is a healthy balance between attachment and exploration. In the insecure-avoidant attachment pattern, a young child turns away or avoids the parent when frightened or in stress. He or she diverts attention instead to exploration. This exploration comes, however, at the expense of the child's attachment needs being met. In the insecure-ambivalent attachment pattern (also called insecure-resistant attachment pattern), the child may seek out the parent for comfort but is highly angry or resistant in the parent's presence. The child cannot be calmed easily and has great difficulties in exploring the environment. A child with an insecure-disorganized attachment pattern has no coherent strategy for seeking out the parent under stress. In infancy, he or she may show overt fear in the parent's presence or show conflicted or disoriented behaviors. Older children with insecure-disorganized attachment show either highly punitive behavior toward their parent under stress or they act as a parent and show caregiving behavior toward their parent under stress. The insecure-disorganized attachment pattern is often seen as a marker for at-risk relationships (Solomon & George, 1999). Table 8.1 links the attachment patterns to parental behaviors that can promote them (Bowlby, 1988; Solomon & George, 1999).

Assessing the various attachment patterns and their manifestations at different developmental periods requires expertise in attachment theory coupled with specialized training. Attachment patterns can be especially difficult to assess if the family has undergone recent disruptions, if the parent has not cared for the child regularly, or if the child has experienced longer separations from the parent (Jacobsen & Miller, 1999).

Other measures can provide rich clinical information on the quality of the parent–child relationship. The CARE-index is an observational measure that assesses both maternal and child behavior based on a brief videotaping of the dyad in a nonstressful situation (Crittenden, 1988, 2001). Raters evaluate a mother's facial expression, vocal expression, position and body contact, expression of affection, pacing, control, and choice of activity. Scoring these behaviors as to their sensitivity can provide information on the overall quality of parenting, ranging from highly sensitive to maltreating parenting. Ratings of children's interactive behavior with their mothers provide information on dimensions of the child's relationship to the mother—the extent to which the child is passive, difficult, or cooperative. Best used with very young children, ratings on the CARE-index have been associated with past child-rearing status (e.g., physically abusive, neglected, marginal, adequate parenting) and with a child's attachment quality to the parent (Crittenden, 1988).

Table 8.1. Attachment patterns and parenting behavior

Attachment pattern	Promoting parental behaviors
Secure	Sensitive and/or responsive parental behavior
Insecure-avoidant	Refusal of child's need for closeness
Insecure-ambivalent	Inconsistent sensitivity to child's needs
Insecure-disorganized	Frightening and/or frightened parental behavior

Measures that provide information on the quality and nature of the parent–child attachment relationship in somewhat older children include an attachment interview for children (Target, Shmueli-Goetz, & Fonagy, 2003), story stems (Hodges, Steele, Hillman, Henderson, & Kaniuk, 2003), narratives (Oppenheim, Emde, & Warren, 1997), and doll play stories that the child enacts (George & Solomon, 1989). In contrast to direct interviews, stories or doll play scenarios may offer children a safe outlet to express their feelings and thoughts about their parent in a context in which there are no real-world consequences (Haight & Miller, 1993).

Observing communication patterns in older children and their parents is another way for clinicians to obtain information on the quality and nature of parent–child attachment relationships. Free-flowing speech between a parent and child coupled with an open discussion of a child's feelings is often indicative of a secure parent–child relationship (Bowlby, 1988). Other positive signs in the parent–child relationship include awareness on the parent and child's part of each other's point of view, goals, feelings, and intentions and an ability to adjust their behavior and negotiate goals through speech. By contrast, long periods of silence and frequent and abrupt topic changes in speech are more common in children who have an insecure attachment quality to their parent (Solomon & George, 1999). How a child and parent talk and respond to each other can reveal other aspects of the relationship quality, including guardedness, poor boundaries, or patterns of blame and anger.

The Separation Anxiety Test assesses children's representations of the self and attachment figures, as well as children's coping abilities based on their responses to imagined parent–child separations (Hansburg, 1972). The child is presented with a series of drawings depicting a variety of situations in which a child experiences a separation, a loss, or the risk of separation or loss. The child is asked whether she has experienced this kind of situation and, if so, how she felt and what she did. A series of follow-up questions are asked about different ways the child in the picture might feel and act. Versions of the test have been linked to behavioral measures of parent–child attachment quality and to measures of children's self-worth (Jacobsen, Edelstein, & Hofmann, 1994).

Assessing the extent to which parent–child interactions are child centered or child directive can provide information on more coercive patterns of parent–child relationships (McMahon & Forehand, 1984). Child-centered interactions include praise, smiles, positive attention, ignoring minor naughtiness, as well as speaking enthusiastically about what the child is saying, doing, or feeling. Child-directive behaviors are negative in nature and include criticism, negative touches, saying "No," teaching, and asking questions. Because no parent is perfect (Winnicott, 1965), it is important to look at the ratio between child-centered and child-directive interactions. An excess of child-directive behaviors is associated with negative child outcomes and with more coercive patterns of parent–child interactions (Patterson, 1982), whereas an excess of child-centered behaviors is linked to more positive child outcomes and better parent–child relationships.

The Attachment Bonds of Children in Foster Care

Assessing the attachment bonds of children in foster care to their biological parents can be a complex task (Jacobsen & Miller, 1999). If the child was removed in infancy and has lived with a foster family for many months, it is likely that the biological parent is not the child's primary attachment figure, although the biological parent may still be an important person in the child's life. If a child is placed in foster care after she has established an attachment bond to the biological parent, the child's feelings and attachment behaviors about the parent can change profoundly during the time the child is in foster care, making it difficult to understand how a particular child feels about his or her parent.

A child who is undergoing a forced separation from a parent may avoid or reject the parent, while also attaching him- or herself with great tenacity to the parent during visits (Bowlby, 1973; Haight, Black, Workman, & Tata, 2001; Robertson & Robertson, 1989). They also may express intense sadness and distress during parent visits. If the child's stay in foster care persists, she may struggle with feelings of conflicting loyalty, especially if the child forms an attachment to the foster parent. If the child is cared for in adverse circumstances (e.g., unstable placement), feelings may be painful to the point that the child responds in an extreme defensive manner when she sees the biological parent. For instance, the child may show little, if any, sign of affection toward the parent during visits (Robertson & Robertson, 1989). Parents are likely to respond to this behavior with anguish.

Children in foster care who have experienced highly aberrant care and/ or frequent disruptions in parenting may show profound and pervasive disturbances in their feelings of security and safety (Zeanah & Boris, 2000). Some indicative signs that a child has developed an atypical or disturbed attachment pattern include a persistent avoidance or gaze aversion of the parent, failure to greet or recognize the parent, a pervasive frustration or anger in the attachment relationship, walking away or sitting with the back to the parent, accident proneness or reckless behavior, self-mutilation, or extreme role reversal (Zeanah et al., 1993).

Clinical attachment disorders involve a serious impairment in a child's ability to trust and to establish a close relationship with an attachment figure (American Psychiatric Association, 2000). Two types of attachment disorders in children are often distinguished: In the first type, the child persistently fails to initiate and respond to social interactions in a developmentally appropriate way. In the second type, the child is indiscriminately friendly toward other adults. In both types, the child fails to form close and meaningful relationships with others.

Sam had been in no less than seven different foster homes by the time he turned 3 years old. When he came in for an assessment, he hugged everyone he met in the waiting room. He asked the clinician who interviewed him whether she could be his mother. Sam also hugged his biological mother after she arrived, but his behavior with her was no different than it was with strangers. Sam's foster father commented on the profound difficulties that Sam had in establishing a meaningful relationship with him, noting, "He doesn't know me from Adam."

Even if a child has a disturbed attachment bond, a parent's behavior toward the child can be telling about the nature of the potential attachment bond that could develop or be re-established between parent and child.

Nelly, a 6-year-old child, had been placed successively in three different foster homes starting when she was 4 years old. In one home, an older foster brother had sexually abused her. When Nelly was observed with her biological mother as part of a parenting assessment, her behavior with her mother was out of control. Nelly became hysterical when she knew that it was time to leave. When her mother tried to hold her, Nelly repeatedly hit her mother while crying. She then banged her head repeatedly on the floor. It was painful for all involved to see the distress that Nelly was experiencing. Nelly's mother remained caring and gentle. She talked calmly with Nelly, reached out and stroked Nelly's cheek and then held her in her arms. Nelly's mother could clearly see how distressed her daughter was, but she tried to reach Nelly emotionally.

If a child is undergoing a prolonged separation from a parent and has lived with foster parents for a longer period of time, the main issue at hand may be to determine who the child's psychological parent is (Goldstein et al., 1998). During a separation, children's behavior toward the biological parent may cool. In some cases, a child may never have had a bond to the parent or the child may have relinquished his or her emotional investment in the parent (Jacobsen & Miller, 1999), especially if the parent does not visit the child regularly or if the separation has been excessively long and stressful. In many instances, children in foster care experience competing loyalties to the biological and foster parents, making it difficult for a clinician to know who the child's psychological parent is.

Phillip, age 8 years, had been living in foster care for a year. His mother had been diagnosed with schizophrenia; his father had a drug addiction. When Phillip arrived at the clinic for an assessment, he was accompanied by his foster parents, who had expressed an interest in adopting him. When Phillip saw his biological parents in the waiting room, he was unable to move toward either set of parents. He looked miserable and was confused about whom he wanted to be with.

Medical, child welfare, and psychological or counseling records can provide a rich source of information that will help an assessor to understand a child's attachment history. The record review should be supplemented with observations of the child with the parent and with interviews of knowledgeable adults (Zeanah & Benoit, 1995). Inquiry is typically made into a child's attachment history about who has cared for the child at different periods of infancy and childhood, how the child has responded to separations, and a child's responses to and behaviors with the parent in attachment situations (e.g., when a child is hurt, frightened, ill; Boris, Fueyo, & Zeanah, 1997). Inquiry should also be made into the quality of care the child has received, including any descriptions of pathogenic care, institutionalization, gross deprivation, or multiple caregivers. The following questions are part of the child's attachment history:

- How long did the child remain with the parent?

- When was the child removed and why?

- Who has the child lived with subsequently?

- What is the child's relationship quality to the parent?

- What is the child's relationship quality to the primary foster caregiver?

- What contact has the child had with the parent?

- How has the child responded to visits?

The Child's Relationships with Others

Looking at the quality of relationships that the child has with other people in his or her life is another important part of the child assessment. Relatives, friends, and other individuals who know the family and child can often compensate for parental mental illness by stepping in to help an ill parent, providing support to the family, and making sure that the child's needs for safety and security are met (Crittenden, 1985). Intimacy and warmth in family relationships can protect a child against stressful life events and provide a child with a more positive outlook and with resolution of day-to-day problems.

The roles of the father, grandparents, or other close relatives are particularly important to examine. The availability of a father and the support received from him can exert a strong impact on a mother and also on child functioning and well-being. If the child's other parent is available and healthy, the child will be less vulnerable to external stressors and mental health problems than if both parents are ill (Rutter, Quinton, & Liddle, 1983).

The child's relationship with siblings is critical to assess. The presence of an older sibling in the family can also make a positive difference for a child growing up in a family with parental mental illness (Göpfert et al., 2004a). However, if there is fragmentation between siblings, resulting conflict and competition may be reinforced, exerting a negative effect on the child's functioning and development (Garcia, Shaw, Winslow, & Yaggi, 2000).

Other adults within the larger family or wider social network can compensate and make a difference by providing support to the parent or child. Relatives who know the child and family may be able to care for a child during a hospitalization or when the parent is unavailable (Smith & Drew, 2002). It is important to keep in mind that the quality of support a child receives is more important than sheer quantity of supports. Therefore, it is essential to ask how committed the person is to the relationship with the child, whether this person can observe and acknowledge risks to the child, and whether this person can intervene on the child's behalf should the situation arise (Göpfert, Webster, & Nelki, 2004b).

Child's Competencies, Coping Skills, and Well-Being

To obtain a rounded picture of the child's overall functioning and well-being and how a mother's mental illness symptoms may have had an impact on it, other aspects of development must be assessed. Which areas to be assessed will depend in part on the child's developmental level and needs, but the areas are likely to include the child's sense of self, her coping skills, and whether the child has behavioral or emotional problems. If the child is in therapy, talking with the treating clinician will be essential. If the child attends school, records or conversations with important teachers may shed light on the child's functioning in this area. This section describes some ways to assess each of these areas.

As noted earlier, children of parents with mental illness are likely to lack confidence in themselves, have low self-esteem, or may have other psychological and behavioral problems. These feelings are often intensified if a child is placed in foster care, where the child is likely to feel grief as well as feelings of helplessness and disempowerment, especially if the child has been excluded from decision making and choices about his or her life (Folman, 1998). Some children may deny symptoms or struggle to share what they experienced at home in an assessment. Others may have been told by parents not to talk about themselves or their lives (Ostler et al., in press).

The hidden nature of the children's problems and the walls of silence that surround them can pose formidable challenges for assessors. Clinicians should, therefore, be aware of the complexities in assessing children's needs and development. Multiple measures, sources, and informants will likely be needed to obtain an accurate picture of children's mental health.

Various measures are available that can provide information on a child's current competencies, coping skills, and sense of self. The Harter's Self Perception Profile (Harter, 1985, 1988) for children, for instance, is a self-report measure that provides information on the child's behavioral conduct, physical appearance, social acceptance, athletic competence, and scholastic competence.

Some measures for older children include the Future Expectations measure (Wyman, Cowen, Work, & Kerley, 1993) and the Can Children Stop Things From Happening? measure (Wannon, 1990). Whereas the Future Expectations measure provides information on what older children think their lives will be like when they grow up and how sure they are of positive outcomes in education, employment, and interpersonal relationships, the Can Children Stop Things from Happening? measure examines the extent to which children can distinguish between events that are controllable and uncontrollable. The latter measure has been found to distinguish children who are resilient and feel they can control events from stress-affected children who feel that events are uncontrollable (Parker, Cowen, Work, & Wyman, 1990).

Determining whether children are experiencing important psychiatric or psychological problems is another area that clinicians will assess when working with a child. Several screening tools can help to screen for such problems. The Children's Depression Scale (Reynolds, 1992) and the Child Depression Inventory (Kovacs, 1985) both provide information on the presence and frequency of depressive symptoms in children. The State-Trait Anxiety Inventory Checklist (Spielberger, 1973) includes questions that ask children to rate how frequently they experience anxiety-related behaviors. The Child Behavior Checklist is a measure of a child's mental health status and is completed by adults who know the child well (Achenbach & Rescorla, 2001). It provides information on externalizing and internalizing symptoms in children and individual scores on eight scales (withdrawn/depressed behavior, somatic complaints, social problems, anxious/depressed behavior, thought problems, attention problems, rule-breaking behavior, aggressive behavior).The Trauma Symptom Checklist for Children (Briere, 1996), another paper and pencil measure, provides information on posttraumatic distress in children who have experienced traumatic events.

As information on a child's development and well-being are gathered, clinicians will also need to establish whether a child's development is atypical and whether the child has special needs. Special needs may include medical, psychiatric, psychological, physical, or educational problems that may require a different standard of parenting. Initial information on a child's special needs can be gathered during the intake process. Doing a record review or talking with the parent often provides information on special needs. Developmental questionnaires can aid in this process as can interviews with the child and with people who know the child well.

Depending on a child's age, several screening tools can provide information on a child's cognitive and linguistic functioning (see Appendix A). If the developmental screening leads a clinician to believe that a child's development or well-being is seriously impaired, then a comprehensive child assessment may be needed to define what interventions will be most helpful to the child. In such circumstances, a clinician may refer the child for a full evaluation.

Finally, to obtain a balanced picture of the child's functioning, attention needs to be given both to a child's strengths and to protective factors in the environment that ameliorate risk (see Table 8.2).

Table 8.2.   Protective factors and strengths

Knowledge that their parent(s) is ill and that they are not to blame
Help and support from family members
A stable home environment
Psychotherapy for the child and the parent(s)
A child's sense of being loved by the ill parent(s)
A naturally stable personality in the child
Positive self-esteem
Inner strength and good coping skills in the child
A strong relationship with a healthy adult
Friendships and positive peer relationships
Interest in and success at school
Healthy interests outside the home for the child
Help from outside the family to improve the family environment
    (e.g., marital psychotherapy, parenting classes)

From American Academy of Child and Adolescent Psychiatry. (2004, July). Facts for families: Children of parents with mental illness. *American Academy of Child and Adolescent Psychiatry, 39*; reprinted by permission.

Synthesizing Findings

In drawing conclusions, the clinician synthesizes what is known about the child's needs, attachment relationships, well-being, and development. It is often helpful to bring a dual lens to this task (Lieberman, Padron, Van Horn, & Harris, 2005). With one lens, the assessor focuses on what the child's experiences have been with his or her family and how the mother's mental illness may have an impact on the particular developmental trajectory this child is taking. Focus is given both to experiences that have introduced unmanageable stress into the child's life and to experiences that may have protected the child (Lieberman et al., 2005). This lens also looks at the role of other important relationships that have made a difference in the child's developmental trajectory.

As the clinician sketches out a working map of the child's experiences, a second lens is used to understand the child's responses to these experiences. This lens focuses on understanding the child's perspective of the parent, her attachment quality, her sense of self and well-being, and her unique areas of resilience and vulnerability across various aspects of development.

By bringing findings from both lenses into clear focus, a clinician can obtain an integrated picture of the child's development, establish what the child's individual needs are, understand what the relationship with the parent means to the child, and determine whether the child's trajectory has been adversely affected by the parent's mental illness. This information will be used in looking at the fit between a parent's skills and the child's needs (Goldstein et al., 1998) and will become part of the written report summarizing the findings on the child. It will also be used in specifying what interventions may help a child (and parent) onto a healthier pathway (Lyons-Ruth et al., 2000).

CONCLUSION

Abundant clinical and observational data indicate that parental mental illness can exert a major impact on a child's well-being and development. Assessing a child's perspectives, needs, and development will be better accomplished if clinicians have a solid understanding of the array of effects that parental mental illness can have on children. The overview and guidelines presented in this chapter were designed to enable clinicians to provide a comprehensive assessment of children who are affected by parental mental illness and to help clinicians to tailor and develop a treatment plan when risk and protective factors for the child's mental health and development are identified.

9

Growing Up Crazy

Niki Grajewski

While teaching a graduate level course on mental disorders at the University of Illinois in Urbana-Champaign, I met Niki, a bright, inquisitive student who always asked relevant and probing questions. After lecturing about how parental mental illness can affect children, Niki came up to me during the break and told me that she knew about bipolar disorder because her mother had been diagnosed with this when she was young. Niki volunteered to talk with the class about her experiences, if I thought it might be helpful.

I asked her how she felt about doing this. She told me it was likely to be hard, but that she had done it before in other classes. It also helped her, she added, whenever she could share her experiences with others. I took Niki up on her offer. The following week, she spoke for about a half hour to the class and then answered questions from her classmates for the next hour. It was a powerful classroom experience for all involved. Initially, the students were silent as Niki told her story, but when she finished, questions poured out and almost everyone participated. I later asked Niki if she would be willing to write a chapter for this book. She agreed immediately.

This chapter describes firsthand what it is like to grow up with a parent who has a chronic mental illness. Niki wrote this chapter as an adult looking back on her years of childhood, adolescence, and early adulthood. Her story illustrates the compassion and love she feels for her mother but also the confusion she felt as a child, her frustration, anger, constant worries, and repeated attempts to do things right. The themes of caring for her mother and parenting a younger sibling are also illustrated in rich detail.

Ultimately, parenting is about parents and about how children fare in their care. This chapter brings the book to a close by presenting in a first-person voice how parental mental illness affects children. It complements Chapter 8, which focuses on how clinicians can assess children's needs, well-being, and development. Having a firm grasp on the variety of outcomes in children, their needs, and their voices is part and parcel of the knowledge base that underlies a sound assessment.

Teresa Ostler

In 4 years I will be 30 years old, the same age that Mom was when she was officially diagnosed with bipolar disorder. To the everyday person, this simply means that I have a mother who is mentally ill, "crazy," and that I am, by mathematical purposes, 26 years old. Although both of these statements are true, they are not the important characteristics about my mom or me. This is purely where we start. What you will find in this account of my life is not in any textbook. This is my real life, that is, how my life has been affected by maternal mental illness.

People often ask me, "When did it all start?" or "When did you know something was wrong?" I don't think I can answer those questions with direct dates or memories. My whole childhood is one blur, with a few happy memories here and there and a whole lot of bad ones that still cloud my mind. When I do talk about how bipolar disorder has affected my life, it often seems jumbled, confusing, and haphazard. For the most part, my life has been all of those things and sometimes still is. However, I will do my best to tell it as it was so that you can see what I went through from day to day. If there is one thing that I have learned from living with mental illness in my family, it is that all anyone can do is his or her best. Even though my mom is mentally ill and some might look at some aspects of her parenting as troubling, I know that with the resources available to her, she did the best that she could.

It is sometimes hard for me to decipher which memories that I have of bad times were the direct result of Mom's mental illness and which were the result of normal stages in my individual and family development. I know that my account is biased in that way. But, being the child of someone who is mentally ill is a special position to be in, and I think my account of what happened has value both for clinicians and for others who have a parent with mental illness.

SOMETHING IS WRONG

Dad was fond of his video camera when we were growing up. He took it everywhere we went. Whether we liked it or not, he tried to record our family memories on tape. I was 6 years old and my sister was 4 when we first started using the video camera. Looking back at those videos, I can now see some of the depression that Mom was experiencing at that time. When Dad could catch Mom on camera, she was usually sullen, shy, and frowning. She hated being taped. When she was on tape, every smile seemed forced.

It was also around age 6 years that I had my first real glimpse at what my mother's illness could do to her and our family. I remember it well: My sister and I are sitting in the bathtub and Mom is cutting our hair. The loose hair on my neck and back itch so badly that all I can do is complain. The next thing I remember is Mom getting frustrated and cutting off our hair.

As a result, both my sister and I ended up looking like boys. Before this, we both had long, beautiful hair.

From then on, things moved pretty fast. We moved from Alaska to Michigan where Dad was being re-stationed in the Army. While he was getting things set up at our new house, we stayed in a little rented apartment in Dad's hometown. When things were good, they were really good, but when things were bad, they sometimes got scary.

While home alone with my mom and sister one day, I remember suddenly being disturbed in play. I looked over to discover that Mom was moaning and crying on the middle of the apartment floor. At this time, I was 7 years old and was already getting used to helping out Mom. But this situation was beyond my control. She was lying on the floor crying and shouting, "I'm going to die, please help me, help me! I'm dying!" For all I knew, she was dying right there in my arms. I was mortified.

This scene went on for half an hour, but in the end I got help from a neighbor. What happened after that is another blur. I know that Mom went to the hospital sometime after that and had gallstones removed. Apparently, they were really painful. It could have been the gallstones that caused Mom to react in such a manner. Maybe her illness symptoms made the display of that pain worse. I am not really sure. But in my young mind, all I felt was that it was my responsibility to do something to help Mom. Thinking back on that incident, I didn't think it was fair, then or now. Little did I know that worrying about Mom's life would become a main part of my life.

The progression of Mom's symptoms became more apparent after this. Not too long after we moved into our new house, my sister and I were shipped to Grandma's house for "a little while." I don't know if either my sister or I had any idea what was going on with Mom at home. Later, I learned that Mom's situation was so bad that my dad ended up calling an ambulance to take her to the hospital. I do know that she was in such a psychotic state that she looked at my dad and saw Jesus looking back at her. Other than that, we never talked about Mom's symptoms or about the other events that led up to that night.

There are a million other small things that Mom did that could have been considered just as strange. Mom never officially worked while she lived with us, but she changed occupations every month or so. She was a pottery and porcelain painter and seller one month, and the next month she was grooming dogs in our garage for the neighbors. Unlike other moms that I knew, Mom was not ashamed of her avid smoking habit, and she did not regularly clean the house.

In the back of my mind, I knew that Mom was exceptional in some way. She was never like my friends' moms, but I accepted that. We rarely got fresh baked cookies or bedtime stories. I always read to myself. For the most part, we had a pretty good family life and enjoyed Mom's spontaneity and sense of fun. When my sister and I moved back home after having lived with Grandma, I hadn't really expected that to change. But it did.

MY "CRAZY" MOM

Because my sister and I were still pretty young, staying at Grandma's for a period of time really didn't mean anything weird to us. We had a great relationship with every member of Dad's family, and spending time with them was enjoyable. One of Dad's sisters returned home to take care of us while Mom was in the hospital.

I really don't know how long we were at Grandma's house or how long Mom stayed in the hospital after we returned home. What I do remember is the private hospital that she stayed in at that time—how it smelled, the fake plants in the huge waiting room, and the line that we stood in to get a soda to drink when we visited her. There were so many rules that I just couldn't understand. Sign in, sign out. How many people will be seeing Mrs. J tonight? How many children? All I knew was that I wanted to see Mom! We frequently visited her with Dad, and the visit was always the same. We sat around a table and tried to find something to say. The sullen, blank stare that my mom often had puzzled me. What did she do all day in this place? When was she coming home? I don't remember saying much during those visits.

One particular visit with Mom has stayed fresh in my mind. We discovered that Mom's doctor had not given permission for children to visit Mom that day. *Children?* Didn't they understand that we weren't just any *children?* Our mom was in there and we wanted to see her. The great solution to this dilemma was for us to go outside of the building and sit on the grass in front of the big window that the hospital cafeteria looked out onto. Mom sat on the other side of the glass and waved.

Even at 8 years old, I knew that this was a raw deal. I have never held back my feelings very well, and, in this instance I didn't either. I threw a fit. I cried. I hid behind a big shrub in the yard because I wasn't going to visit Mom through a window! In the end, I joined my dad and sister at the window, but I don't think I waved or tried to communicate with Mom. No matter what circumstances we were in, Mom was always happy to see us, and she always let us know that she loved us. Even through a big window, you could tell this just by looking at her. She might be crazy, but she loved us dearly.

Eventually, Mom returned home with loads of pills and one of those seven-day plastic medicine containers. Our aunt left, and life continued. Mom smoked her cigarettes and drank Pepsi with a passion, and my sister and I pretty much did whatever we wanted to do. Mom had good days and bad, but things were never normal. Laughing at inappropriate moments was common for Mom to do. But that laugh is still precious to me. I can hear it in my mind, and it makes me smile. Her laughter and comical nature are infectious, and to this day, I don't think she has a hard time making friends.

Sometimes the poor judgment that the illness seemed to bring out in Mom brought us a lot of unexpected pleasure. Twice we came home from school to find Mom sitting in our yard with a new dog. So what if one of the dogs cost $500? I don't think that Dad had a part in the decision. But he always let these things slide. Those two dogs stayed in our family until one passed away and the other was given to a loving family when my dad could no longer care for it. Times like those—getting a new job, a shopping spree, a surprise here and there—were fun for us. They also provided an escape from the times that were bad.

Once, Mom took us to a huge dog show in Detroit, and just because she thought it would be fun, she snuck our puppy inside the venue in her coat. I remember telling her, "No, Mom, we can't do that. Read the sign, 'No outside dogs allowed.'" Whenever I would try to point out the obvious wrongdoing of her behavior, she would just chuckle and continue on her way.

It is important to note that while Mom was still living with us, my sister and I rarely saw her in a manic state. It was as if Dad and Mom could see it coming. Before we knew it, Mom would be back in the hospital. To me, the hospital only made things worse for her. Mom started to take up relationships with other men in the psychiatric ward. I remember her telling me that she told one man that she was married but that she didn't care. I could never understand this. Dad was the most loving, supportive man and did everything in his power to help Mom. He also did everything to make things right for us, regardless of our problems. I have a picture of Mom and Dad hugging outside of the hospital when she got released one time. For some reason, I still love that picture. It shows my dad's undying support and love for Mom, when I know she was so hard to live with.

After Mom attempted to file for divorce, took it back, filed again, and then rescinded it, Dad had had enough. My parents decided to separate. When Mom told me that they were separating, I was devastated. I was so sure that divorce could never happen to my family. Mom didn't leave right away, either. She came and went whenever she pleased for some time. There were several other events that led up to Dad's decision to obtain a divorce.

Picture this: I come home from school with a girlfriend one day. I'm 12 years old. There is a note on the coffee table, but no one else is home. The note read something like this, "I'm sorry. I just can't take the weather any more. I have gone to Florida with Sara [fake name given to protect my sister] and Rascal [one of the dogs]. Mom." My mouth gaped open for at least 2 minutes. I was lucky that I had a supportive friend with me that day. Dad was not due home for hours, and I was thunderstruck. I had not been witness to anything like this before.

Amazingly, Dad did very little to stop her apparent move to Florida with my sister but rode the waves of what this seemingly manic episode was doing to our family. In those days, I stuck to my friends for dear life, went to church, and clung to Dad. Mom even enrolled my sister in school in Florida, and I was certain that we had lost them both forever. Eventually, Mom called Dad from some hospital in Kentucky or Tennessee, where she had checked herself in. Dad drove down there to get Mom and my sister, who waited for more than 7 hours in the hospital waiting room. She was probably only 9 years old at the time.

When Mom left for Florida, she wiped out our family savings accounts and maxed out our credit cards. Living in the military, we never had very much to begin with, but Mom took it all. When I found out that Dad had decided to get a divorce, and I knew that he was the one to initiate and complete all of the legal work to end the marriage, I was mad at him. At times, I even think I went so far as to "hate" him. Now, I understand that he did all that he could for Mom and all that he could to keep the family together. He tried his best. I'm still not certain why he did divorce Mom, but the financial insecurity that the illness brought to our family and the possible danger that it brought to us kids were probably weighing heavily on his mind.

My family experience is filled with so much silence and denial that even today I am baffled by how much we managed to *not* talk about what was going on. Of all of us, I am the most verbal. But even I was pretty silent on issues regarding Mom's bipolar disorder. That is just the way that I learned to deal with her illness. To keep things inside is more painful than hiding the deepest and darkest secret. My sister, dad, and I never sat down to talk about what was happening to Mom or to discuss things that made no sense but that affected us all, like the abrupt move to Florida. I'm not sure that the way we dealt with Mom's illness was necessarily right or wrong. For the most part it seemed to work for us. But in keeping silent about my mom's illness, we alienated her as a person. We didn't try to understand or contemplate what the illness was doing to her. For all I knew at that time, I just had a mom who was "crazy."

We alienated Mom in such a way that she became this woman whom none of us wanted to talk to, be around, or think about. Her actions and feelings permeated our whole lives. Because we mainly saw her as being mentally ill, we chalked up all of her as being mentally ill, as well. In a sense, her name changed from Ann to "that mentally ill woman." It was hard for us to accept her then, but it is even harder for me now to accept the way our whole family treated her back then.

PARENTING THE PARENT

After Mom was diagnosed and came home from the hospital, her role as a parent changed. At this time, I was 8 years old and my sister was about 6. Mom still cooked us meals and kept the house relatively clean, but more and more I found myself taking on additional responsibilities. Even prior to her illness, I had always volunteered to do chores around the house, but in the years following her hospitalization I found out that if I didn't do things around the house, they just never got done. If I didn't volunteer to dust, a film would begin to collect on our furniture. I began to help with the laundry and clean the house. This may sound normal for a 10-year-old child, but the level of responsibility that I began to assume was, in my eyes, inappropriate.

Picture this scene: Mom is standing in the doorway to my sister's room and is yelling at her. I come out of my room to see what is going on. My sister is just standing there wide-eyed. Mom has grabbed her arm and is about to hit her.

"Mom! No! Stop it!" Mom looks at me, looks at my sister, runs to her room, and slams the door. You can hear her crying down the hall. I go into her room and she is sobbing on the bed with her hands over her face.

"I'm a horrible mom! I'm a horrible mom! I don't deserve to live! I'm sorry! I'm sorry!" I automatically go to her side and console her. I rub her back and tell her that she isn't a horrible mom and that it's all okay. I am 12 years old.

My parents had never spanked us or disciplined us physically. So seeing Mom about to hit my little sister took me by surprise. We were not perfect children, but for some reason I knew that whatever my sister had done, she hadn't deserved Mom's grabbing and hitting her. I never found out why Mom was about to hit my sister, and we never talked about it afterward, but the incident still stands out in my mind. The scene of Mom becoming upset and me consoling her became a regular pattern in our lives. Until I moved too far away to be a physical presence for Mom, I was always her consoler.

Around the same time, I became overly protective of my sister. We fought like dogs at home and were often mean to each other, but if someone outside of our family was mean to my sister, I became enraged. I am still protective of her and often think of her as my child. When she entered puberty, I was the one who explained puberty to her. When she needed clothes or help with hygiene, I was the one who dealt with the situation. Due to the helping nature of my character, I didn't mind this role very much, but it was still hard for both my sister and me to understand why Mom wasn't present.

My sister and I are only about 2 years apart in age, but it seemed like we were far apart when it came to maturity and overall development. I can't count how many times I fought with my sister to brush her teeth, take a shower, or brush her hair. When she went to her senior prom, I came home from college so that I could help her with her hair and makeup. I love that girl so much that it brings tears to my eyes. I feel more sadness about the problems she has suffered due to our family circumstances than I feel about my own suffering.

After Mom and Dad divorced and Mom moved out, the responsibility that I had for Mom became even more demanding. It was not uncommon for me to get a message over the high-school loud speaker telling me that I had a phone call. It was always Mom asking for a ride here or there or asking me to come and get her out of some troubling situation. *In the middle of high school!* Eventually, I had to have Dad call the school and inform them not to accept any phone calls from Mom. It seemed that no matter where I was, Mom found a way to engage me in her problems. I couldn't find respite anywhere.

There were countless instances when I came to Mom's rescue, but two stand out. The first instance occurred when I was still in high school. Mom called me at 11 at night and asked me to pick her up at a local bowling alley. I was caught off-guard because I had thought that my mom was living in Florida. But she was in town. When she called, she told me that all I had to do was to drive her to a friend's house. Although it was already late in the evening, I managed to get a friend to drive with me to the bowling alley. But when I went inside, I could not find Mom anywhere. I asked the attendant, but no one had seen her. My friend and I returned to the car and sat there for a few minutes while I tried to decide what to do. After a few moments, what looked like a skinny old man came running toward my car. Mom's face appeared in my driver's window. My heart raced. Her hair was so short she looked like a man and she was skinnier than I had ever seen her. She insisted that we leave immediately, so my friend got in the back and Mom took the passenger seat. When I asked her where her friend lived, she said that she wasn't sure. When I asked her if she could call her friend, she said she didn't know the number. Finally, she admitted that she never intended to go to a friend's house but just wanted me to come pick her up.

By that time, I could tell that Mom was in a manic state. Her thoughts were racing. She was fidgeting and displaying paranoia by looking around with a terrified look on her face. Mom yelled at me, and then almost broke down in tears. As I drove around, she proceeded to tell me that while she was in Florida, the government found out that she knew about a secret plot to drug everybody in the country by putting poison in our food sources. According to Mom, the government found out that she knew and wanted to kill her.

At that time, Mom was so skinny because she was afraid that the government would know where she was and what she ate. She was also convinced they would poison her. So the move from Florida to Michigan was due to the government chasing her and to Mom not knowing where else to go. While Mom was telling me this story, she was crouched down on the floor of the passenger seat, afraid that "they" would see her.

I had no idea what to do. As a 17-year-old, all I could think of was, *this is not my job!* I was also embarrassed that my friend was witnessing this scene. After driving around for what seemed like an eternity, Mom finally told me to drop her off at the downtown Detroit bus station. If you have ever been to the bus station in downtown Detroit, you would have been as afraid and discouraged as I was at that moment. I knew that I had no choice. I had no money for a hotel. Dad wasn't home when I left, and I didn't want to bother him with Mom and her problems anyway. I couldn't bring her back to Dad's house; it just didn't seem right. So I made my way to the bus station in the middle of the night.

Mom had not eaten in who knows how long, and I couldn't just leave her in the bus station. I scrounged up some loose change and bought her some food from a vending machine. Surprisingly, she ate it. It was raining outside and Mom was soaked, so I also gave her my coat and the shoes off my feet. That night I gave her everything that I had. I gave her everything and more. I had to leave her there with all of the other homeless men and women, including those who wanted us to buy dope and those who were sleeping on the benches.

I cried the whole way home. The feelings that I had are similar to what I feel whenever I spend time with Mom. Guilt for all that I had and all that she never would have fills me to the brim to this day. I feel a great sadness for all the hardship that she has had to endure. I also felt anger toward Mom. Sometimes I blamed her for the situations that she got herself into, and sometimes I just needed to be angry at someone—she was an easy target. I also felt a fair degree of hopelessness. No matter what I did for her, it never seemed like it would be enough to make her better or to improve her life.

The second instance that stands out in my mind occurred when I was on college break. At that time, I was receiving specialized training in my hometown to become a direct-care worker. This means I was beginning a job at a group home caring for adults with developmental delays. I didn't know it, but the building where I was doing my training was the same mental health center where Mom was seeing a counselor. During a lunch break with a friend, I suddenly saw Mom talking with another classmate of mine. Again, I could immediately see that Mom was in a manic state. When she saw me, she rambled and complained. She told me that she was pissed off and depressed and that no one would do anything to help her.

I asked Mom why she was there, and she said her counselor worked in the building. She was trying to see him. The building was situated on a four-lane street, and Mom was threatening to run into the street and kill herself. I finally understood: Mom had been trying to see her counselor but had been turned away.

I went up to the receptionist to see if I could help Mom see her counselor. I was turned away. The reason I was given was that Mom did not have an appointment. Moreover, her counselor did not have time to see her. While I was talking to the receptionist, Mom ran around the building and threatened to run into the street. One of my friends was chasing her. Finally, we got Mom into the lobby bathroom. There, Mom paced around while my friend stood guard at the door. I, in turn, argued with the receptionist. The scene was totally chaotic. Other patients told the receptionist that Mom could go in before them. In the meantime, Mom became more and more anxious and angry. I, too, found myself feeling angry and anxious. Before I realized what I was doing, I found myself punching the receptionist's window out of frustration.

When the receptionist came to the window, she informed me that Mom's counselor would like to talk to me before he talked with Mom. This confused me. Mom was the one who was threatening suicide and running around the building, and I was the one he chose to talk to. When I went into his office, the therapist jumped right into telling me that my mom was the most manipulative woman in the county, and that I had to stop enabling her. I was flabbergasted! I just didn't want her to kill herself; I didn't know that what I was doing was called "enabling." The therapist also told me that it wasn't my job to take care of my mom and that I had to live my own life. I knew all of the things he was telling me were true, and others will probably agree with his statements. But at that time, I felt like I held Mom's life in my hands, and I was going to do anything I could to continue her life. *That* is over-responsibility.

Although I sometimes was resentful of all that I did for Mom, I feel that if I had not done those things for her, no one else would have stepped in to help. Her family ignored her emotional needs and denied that she was mentally ill. She was not allowed to stay at their houses or to attend holiday gatherings. I am and always have been her main family support system. She often tells me not to act like her mother, but I feel that is a role that she unknowingly asked me to fill long ago. I also feel that I can't give up on her.

"I MUST BE CRAZY, TOO"

After telling other people about my experiences with Mom's bipolar disorder, they are amazed at how well I have turned out. People also tell me how well I have managed to separate myself from the experiences related to Mom's illness. I'm still not sure that either of these observations is completely accurate. Ever since I was old enough to actually realize that the mental illness my mom had was serious and pervasive, it has taken a hold of my life in an awkward way. Yes, I can talk about it objectively, but does it still affect me now as it did when I was 12? You bet ya.

At a pretty young age, I started to see that what was going on in my family was anything but normal. When my parents decided to separate, it hit me pretty hard, and I'm not sure I managed to pick myself up completely until about 3 years ago. I'm 26 now and was 12 then. The mathematics of all of those years that I viewed myself as someone in crisis are important because no matter how resilient people might view me as being today, I experienced a lot of pain growing into the person who I am now. No matter how proud and pleasantly surprised I am that I have made it this far, I would have rather done without all of the hardship that I had to go through.

At one point in my life, I never thought that I would make it as far as I have. Before I finished high school, I had the idea set in my mind that I would never make it to see my 21st birthday. There were many things that led me to believe this. By the time I was 13, I was a regular self-cutter. This meant that when times got rough, I found whatever object I could to harm myself. In junior high, I even used a staple to cut my hand. That action totally caught me off-guard. It also embarrassed the friends who watched me do it.

We were playing some dare game, and one of my girlfriends dared another, "I bet you can't cut yourself with a staple!" The girl who was dared did not cut herself; she couldn't do it. "Oh, yeah, well I can do it, no problem," I said. And I did cut myself with that staple, for no reason other than to prove that I was tough. It was a minor cut and barely drew any blood. At this point in my life, I don't remember that it caused any pain. However, at that time I did it because deep inside I enjoyed causing myself pain. It was a way to release some of the pent-up rage, sadness, and despair that was becoming a regular part of my life. The next year in junior high, I used an eraser to burn into my thigh "I 'heart' W.R." (These were the initials of a guy that I was "madly in love with.") I did this while my math teacher was talking about algebraic equations. One of my friends looked on at me in awe. The scar stood about four inches tall and three inches wide. It only started to completely fade away a couple of years ago.

This pattern of cutting, hurting, and scarring myself continued until I was an undergraduate in college. Sometimes I used dull scissors and sometimes I used erasers. The wounds were never deep enough to cause serious harm, but they were plentiful. When I couldn't bear to make myself bleed, I banged my head against something or punched my thighs and stomach with my fists. Like most people who cut, I did these things to give myself some release from the emotional pain that I was feeling. My sadness ran so deep, and I cried so much inside. I guess causing myself pain gave me something else to cry about. Sometimes I did these things alone in my room before I went to bed, and sometimes I did them in front of other people.

To replace the love that I somehow felt that I lost when my parents divorced, I became obsessed with boys to an extreme degree. If a boy I liked didn't call me or talk to me at school, I would cry uncontrollably, hurt myself, and fall asleep in tears. One Friday night at the local bowling alley, I became extremely distraught when the boy whose initials I had carved into my leg 2 years earlier showed interest in one of my best friends. I went out to my car in the parking lot and just lost it. I started to cry and wail and locked myself in my car. Some of my friends came out looking for me and tried to get me to come out, but I just couldn't. I felt as though no one cared about me or my feelings, and I also felt completely out of control. Banging my head on the steering wheel didn't seem to help, but I did it anyway. I also banged my wrists on the steering wheel and then banged my head against the window. I'm not sure how long this went on, but I eventually let a friend in the car, and she talked me into going back into the bowling alley. By then, most people who knew me recognized that at times I could be unstable, but luckily my friends never completely shied away from me or my problems.

When I wasn't acting as though I was off my rocker, I did have a lot of friends and acquaintances who helped to fill in time. For most of high school, filling in time was essential for getting me through. In my eyes, high school was a war zone, with nothing but heartache for me to experience. Up until that point in my life, with everything that I had experienced, the memories that I had were painful. I felt destined to lead a doomed life.

I played three sports each year until I was a senior in high school. I worked part time and spent the rest of my time with friends. If you asked those friends what kind of friend I was, they would probably say that I was "nice" . . . overly nice, if you ask me. It could have been my need for acceptance and approval, but I can remember doing anything that my friends asked me to do, at any time. I was the go-to person. When my friends had problems, they came to me. I enjoyed this immensely, and I reveled in the attention that this somehow brought me. I liked to make other people happy, even if I could do nothing to make myself feel any real joy.

I was, and still am, a classic overachiever. I got straight As, was in the honor society, and was every teacher's favorite pupil. The last 2 years of high school, I added karate to my daily routine, and by the time I went to college, I had already gotten my brown belt. So you may be thinking, "Wow," "Great," or "Good for her," but this cycle of constantly striving to be perfect at everything also caused me grief. When I was a freshman basketball player, I would go into hysterics if we lost a game. My coach at the time used to tell me that if I didn't lighten up, I would have a heart attack before I graduated. During classes, if I got anything lower than an A, I would cry. Any type of failure was catastrophic to me. My dad never drove my sister and me hard, and there was no outside pressure for me to do well at anything. All of the pressure to do well came from me.

During the time I attended high school, I still experienced crying spells that I couldn't control. Luckily, I had a teacher, who was also my coach and friend, who allowed me to sit in her office to pull myself together. I could get a pass from another teacher and go to my coach, and she would allow me to skip the next hour and a half of classes just so I could get away. At this time, I also developed troubling stomachaches and pains that would often take me out of class. Later, I learned that I had Irritable Bowel Syndrome which, not surprisingly, is often caused by stress.

Throughout my life, I have struggled with issues relating to body image. Starting when I was 12 years old, I would try anything I could to lose weight. I started stealing laxatives, taking mini-thins, starving myself, and purging. I still have some problems with weight issues, but I no longer engage in negative behaviors. The issues with weight had a lot to do with an unhealthy lifestyle growing up and a slight weight problem, but now I think that trying to control my weight was another issue of control. Just as cutting or hurting myself was an issue of control, binging and purging was an issue of control. My life seemed so chaotic and out of control that those negative behaviors allowed me to control something in my life. I still do not think that either of my parents know that I had these problems.

When I first started cutting, Mom and Dad did notice the carved initials in my leg. Mom even attempted to take me to see a child psychiatrist. She made the appointment and took me out of school for the day. To butter me up to the idea, she took me shopping before the appointment. After she bought me what I wanted, I told her that I really didn't want to go to see a child psychiatrist, insisting that I was fine. Without an argument at all, Mom took me home and forgot about the appointment altogether.

There are only two other times that I talked to a mental health professional about the depression and other mental health problems that I was experiencing. The first was with a high-school counselor whom I asked to see because I was having serious thoughts of suicide. The main things that I remember from those eight short sessions are crying a lot and the counselor telling me in the final session that she could no longer see me and that she wished me well. I was devastated, angry, and even more depressed that when I finally sought help, I was basically turned away.

The only other time that I spoke to a mental health professional was at my own request. I asked my dad to take me to talk to someone. I was again depressed, suicidal, and feeling that I could no longer handle the stress in my life. My dad took me to see a child psychiatrist who placed a box of Kleenex in my lap and listened to me cry for an hour as I tried to tell her my worries. Going to see the psychiatrist was like an act of admission to me. I was admitting that I was messed up like my mom. And although I knew that I was feeling horribly and did need help, I didn't want to be labeled. Diagnosed. I didn't want to cry about it and have people feel sorry for me. And that is what I thought would happen: I would cry, the psychiatrist would label me, medicate me, and I would become "crazy." The experience was horrible for me, and afterward I told my dad that I didn't want to go back. He never made me go again.

I do not blame my parents for not making me attend counseling. My parents were unaware of half of the things I was going through. They were dealing with their own stress and had to take care of themselves and my little sister. I know that my dad did the best that he could. Being a single father with two girls and an ex-wife with bipolar disorder who was a constant presence in our lives could not have been easy. Without him being strong and supporting my sister and me, we might not be as healthy and stable as we both are today.

Today, my dad, sister, and I are closer than ever. When Mom calls me, I often call Dad just to vent about the stress her phone calls bring me. I just want him to tell me that it's not my job to take care of her. He still sends her alimony checks, but she knows that she cannot manipulate him any longer. Sometimes my husband will tell her I'm not home when she calls. My family talks about the past more, but we no longer let it consume us. We know that Mom is mentally ill—she does some things she shouldn't—but we try not to hold it against her. We ride the waves when they come, and try to return to some sort of normalcy in our own lives.

IF ONLY. . .

I have never been a fan of statements that start with the words "if only. . . ." I could fill a million pages of "if onlys" that would have made all of our lives better. I am sad that we had to experience all of the negative things that we did, but I do not regret having had them. Those experiences have helped to shape me into the person I am today, and I would not take back the experiences I had. We played with the cards that we were dealt and came out winners overall. However, there are some things that I have thought about that could have been helpful to my family and me along the way.

There were many times that I would go with Mom to her counseling appointments and wait for her in the waiting room. Even though I was a young child when my mom was first diagnosed, I would have appreciated an explanation about why my mom was changing before my eyes. My parents did not talk to my sister and me about Mom's illness, but it might have helped us to conceptualize what was happening. So many people told me that because my mom had bipolar disorder, I would also become ill. It was not until college that I heard that environmental factors also can play into the development of some mental illnesses.

It would have been helpful for my whole family and me to attend some sort of family counseling or support group. We all managed, but it was probably not the healthiest environment for any of us. Again, we did the best that we could, but any help to support us in our lives would have been appreciated. Family counseling or support would have been helpful to assist us in the adjustment to parental divorce and the switch in roles that we all undertook as a result of this. It would have also helped us to function as a loving family through all of our problems.

I felt so isolated being a child of someone who was mentally ill. It was, and still sometimes is, a deep dark secret that I keep inside. It is a secret that eats away at my heart, my mind, and my soul. If I would have known other children who were also experiencing some of the same things I was, it would have been such a relief to me. Now when I meet people who disclose that they have a parent or a relative who is mentally ill, it sheds a small ray of light on my heart. I am not alone. Other children who have a parent or relative that is mentally ill are not alone. We should not have to feel that way, and if anything can be done to bring those suffering together and to break down the sense of loneliness and isolation that results from silence, it would greatly assist in healthy growth, high self-esteem, and wellness.

When I start to remember things that have happened in my life and the craziness that we dealt with, I wonder if people will even believe half of the stories I tell. This is what happened in my family from my point of view, the point of view of a child. It hurts me to retell these stories, but it is what it is, and I am proud to be able to tell the stories. My mom still has problems that may be associated with her mental illness, and I still try to support her in any way that I can.

I have not seen Mom in almost 5 years, and my sister hasn't seen her for an even longer period of time. Mom has yet to meet my husband. I am still scared for my 30th birthday, the age when Mom was diagnosed with bipolar disorder. I know that if I can make it this far, I can make it through anything, but that does not make dealing with Mom's illness any easier. I might be successful, healthy, and happy, but I think about Mom every day. I am scared for her every day. I am scared for me and my sister every day, too. However, we have made it this far, and I have hope for and confidence in all of us. We may all have been resilient, but we still have pain.

I still have never participated in any counseling or therapy. I am proud of how far I feel that I have come emotionally, mentally, and physically. Attending counseling or therapy might have made a difference, especially with the many transitions I went through. I guess I am still just as afraid as I was as an adolescent of the stigma that surrounds mental illness and of being labeled, due to my mom being sick. What I know now that would have been helpful to me, and will be helpful to other children of mentally ill parents, is that my feelings were normal for the circumstances I was in. To some extent, I had choices about how my life turned out. I no longer feel doomed to have a hard life, and other children should not feel that way, either. What I needed growing up—what all children need—was support, empathy, understanding, love, and people to have faith in me that I could overcome my obstacles.

The problems that families who encounter mental illness may face are vast. The surface picture does not always present a clear picture of what the experience is like for every member of the family. Look deep. Look hard. Pay attention to the small details. Please do not assume that just because a parent is mentally ill, it means that he or she cannot care for or love his or her children. Please do not assume that just because a parent is mentally ill, it means that his or her children are, too. I know that my mom was far from perfect, but I am still glad that she was a part of my life. As strange as that sounds, I am. There is love behind the mask of mental illness. There is also hope.

References

Abernathy, V.D., & Grunebaum, H.L. (1972). Toward a family planning program in psychiatric hospitals. *American Journal of Public Health, 62,* 1638–1645.

Abidin, R.R. (1990). *Parenting Stress Index* (short form). Charlottesville, VA: Pediatric Psychology Press.

Achenbach, T.M., & Rescorla, L.A. (2001). *Manual for the ASEBA School-Age Forms & Profiles.* Burlington: University of Vermont, Research Center for Children, Youth, & Families.

Ackerson, B.J. (2003). Coping with the dual demands of severe mental illness and parenting: The parent's perspective. *Families in Society: The Journal of Contemporary Human Services, 84,* 109–118.

Adshead, G., Falkov, A., & Göpfert, M. (2004). Personality disorder in parents: Developmental perspectives and intervention. In M. Göpfert, J. Webster, & M.V. Seeman (Eds.), *Parental psychiatric disorder* (2nd ed., pp. 217–240). Cambridge, MA: Cambridge University Press.

Ainsworth, M.D.S., Blehar, M.C., Waters, E., & Wall, S. (1978). *Patterns of attachment: A psychological study of the strange situation.* Hillsdale, NJ: Lawrence Erlbaum Associates.

Alpern, L., & Lyons-Ruth, K. (1993). Preschool children at social risk: Chronicity and timing of maternal depressive symptoms and child behavior problems at school and at home. *Development and Psychopathology, 5,* 371–387.

Altshuler, L.L., & Kiriakos, C. (2006). Bipolar disorder: Special issues in pregnancy and the postpartum. In V. Hendrick (Ed.), *Current clinical practice: Psychiatric disorders in pregnancy and the postpartum: Principles and treatment* (pp. 109–138). Totowa, NJ: Humana Press.

Amador, X.F., Strauss, D.H., Yale, S.A., & Gorman, J.M. (1991). Awareness of illness in schizophrenia. *Schizophrenia Bulletin, 17,* 113–132.

American Academy of Child and Adolescent Psychiatry. (2004, July). *Facts for families: Children of parents with mental illness. American Academy of Child and Adolescent Psychiatry* (No. 39). Retrieved from http://aacap.org/page.ww?name = Children + of + Parents + with + Mental + Illness&section = Facts + for + Families

American Psychiatric Association. (2000). *Diagnostic and statistical manual of mental disorders* (4th ed., text rev.). Washington, DC: Author.

American Psychological Association. (2001). *Empirical studies on gay and lesbian parenting.* Retrieved March 19, 2004, from http://www.apa.org/pi/l&gbib.html

Anthony, E.J. (1971). Folie à deux: A developmental failure in the process of separation-individuation. In J.B. McDevitt & C.F. Settlage (Eds.), *Separation-individuation: Essays in honor of Margaret S. Mahler* (pp. 253–273). New York: International Universities Press.

Apfel, R.J., & Handel, M.H. (1993). *Madness and loss of motherhood: Sexuality, reproduction, and long-term mental illness.* Washington, DC: American Psychiatric Press.

Appleby, L., & Dickens, C. (1993). Mothering skills of women with mental illness. *British Medical Journal, 306,* 348–349.

Arnold, D.S., O'Leary, S.G., Wolff, L.S., & Acker, M.M. (1993). The parenting scale: A measure of dysfunctional parenting in discipline situations. *Psychological Assessment, 5,* 137–144.

Azar, S.T., Lauretti, A.F., & Loding, B.V. (1998). The evaluation of parental fitness in termination of parental rights cases: A functional-contextual perspective. *Clinical Child and Family Psychology Review, 1,* 77–100.

Azar, S.T., Povilaitis, T.Y., Lauretti, A.F., & Pouquette, C.L. (1998). The current status of etiological theories in intrafamilial child maltreatment. In J.R. Lutzker (Ed.), *Handbook of child abuse research and treatment* (pp. 3–30). New York: Plenum Press.

Azar, S.T., Robinson, D.R., Hekimian, E., & Twentyman, C.T. (1984). Unrealistic expectations and problem solving ability in maltreating and comparison mothers. *Journal of Consulting and Clinical Psychology, 52,* 687–691.

Baker, P.L., & Carson, A. (1999). "I take care of my kids": Mother practices of substance-abusing women. *Gender & Society, 13,* 347–363.

Barnum, R. (1997). A suggested framework for forensic consultation in cases of child abuse and neglect. *The Journal of the American Academy of Psychiatry and the Law, 25,* 581–593.

Barrera, I. (2003). From rocks to diamonds: Mining the riches of diversity for our children. *Zero to Three, 23*(5), 8–15.

Barrera, M., Jr. (1981). Social support in the adjustment of pregnant adolescents: Assessment issues. In B.H. Gottlieb (Ed.), *Social networks and social support* (pp. 69–96). Beverly Hills, CA: Sage Publications.

Battaglia, J. (2001, October 11). Compliance with treatment in schizophrenia. Retrieved November 11, 2001, from http://psychiatry.medscape.com/Medscape/CNO/2001/apaips/Story.cfm?

Bavolek, S.J. (1987). Adult Adolescent Parenting Inventory (AAPI). In K. Corcoran & J. Fischer (Eds.), *Measures for clinical practice: A sourcebook* (pp. 415–418). New York: Free Press.

Bavolek, S.J. (2000). Adult-Adolescent Parenting Inventory (AAPI). In K. Corcoran & J. Fischer (Eds.), *Measures for clinical practice: A sourcebook: Vol.1. Couples, families, and children* (pp. 204–206). New York: Free Press.

Bavolek, S.J., Kline, D., & McLaughlin, J. (1979). Primary prevention of child abuse: Identification of high risk adolescents. *Child Abuse and Neglect: The International Journal, 3,* 1071–1080.

Beardslee, W.R., Versage, E.M., & Gladstone, T.R.G. (1998). Children of affectively ill parents: A review of the past 10 years. *Journal of the American Academy of Child and Adolescent Psychiatry, 37,* 1134–1141.

Belsky, J. (1980). Child maltreatment: An ecological integration. *American Psychologist, 35,* 320–335.

Belsky, J. (1984). The determinants of parenting: A process model. *Child Development, 55,* 83–96.

Belsky, J. (1993). Etiology of child maltreatment: A developmental-ecological analysis. *Psychological Bulletin, 114,* 413–434.

Benjamin, L.R., Benjamin, R., & Rind, B. (1996). Dissociative mothers' subjective experiences of parenting. *Child Abuse and Neglect: The International Journal, 20,* 933–942.

Berg-Nielsen, T.S., Vikan, A., & Dahl, A. (2002). Parenting related to child and parental psychopathology: A descriptive review of the literature. *Clinical Child Psychology and Psychiatry, 7,* 529–552.

Besinger, B.A., Garland, A.F., Litrownik, A.J., & Landsverk, J.A. (1999). Caregiver substance abuse among maltreated children placed in out-of-home care. *Child Welfare, 78,* 221–239.

Bifulco, A., Brown, G.W., & Harris, T.O. (1994). Childhood Experience of Care and Abuse (CECA): A retrospective interview measure. *Journal of Child Psychology and Psychiatry and Applied Disciplines, 35,* 1419–1435.

Bifulco, A., Moran, P., Ball, C., & Bernazzani, O. (2002). Adult attachment style: Its relationship to clinical depression. *Social Psychiatry and Psychiatric Epidemiology, 37,* 50–59.

Blanch, A.K., Nicholson, J., & Purcell, J. (1994). Parents with severe mental illness and their children: The need for human services integration. *Journal of Mental Health Administration, 21,* 388–396.

Bloom, H., Webster, C., Hucker, S., & De Freitas, K. (2005). The Canadian contribution to violence risk assessment: History and implications for current psychiatric practice. *Canadian Journal of Psychiatry, 50,* 3–11.

Boris, N.W., Fueyo, M., & Zeanah, C.H. (1997). The clinical assessment of attachment in children under five. *Journal of the American Academy of Child and Adolescent Psychiatry, 36,* 291–293.

Boris, N.W., Wheeler, E.E., Heller, S.S., & Zeanah, C.H. (2000). Attachment and developmental psychopathology, *Psychiatry, 63,* 75–84.

Bowlby, J. (1973). *Attachment and loss, volume II: Separation: Anxiety and anger.* New York: Basic Books.

Bowlby, J. (1988). *A secure base: Clinical applications of attachment theory.* London: Routledge.

Briere, J. (1996). *Trauma Symptom Checklist for Children (TSCC): Professional manual.* Odessa, FL: Psychological Assessment Resources.

Briggs, H.E., & Rzepnicki, T.L. (Eds.). (2004). *Using evidence in social work practice: Behavioral perspectives.* Chicago: Lyceum Books.

Brodzinsky, D.M. (1993). On the use and misuse of psychological testing in child custody evaluations. *Professional Psychology: Research and Practice, 24,* 213–219.

Brunette, M., & Jacobsen, T. (2006). Children of parents with mental illness: Outcomes and interventions. In V. Hendrick (Ed.), *Current clinical practice: Treatment of psychiatric disorders in pregnancy and the postpartum: Principles and treatment* (pp. 197–227). Totowa, NJ: Humana Press.

Budd, K.S., & Holdsworth, M.J. (1996). Methodological issues in assessing minimal parenting competency. *Journal of Clinical Child Psychology, 25,* 2–14.

Budd, K.S., Poindexter, L.M., Felix, E.D., & Naik-Polan, A.T. (2001). Clinical assessment of parents in child protection cases: An empirical analysis. *Law and Human Behavior, 25,* 93–108.

Burton, Jr., V.S. (1990). The consequences of official labels: A research note on rights lost by the mentally ill, mentally incompetent, and convicted felons. *Community Mental Health Journal, 26,* 267–276.

ByBee, D., Mowbray, C.T., Oyserman, D., & Lewandowski, L. (2003, July–September). Variability in community functioning of mothers with serious mental illness. *The Journal of Behavioral Health Services & Research, 30,* 269–289.

Byng-Hall, J. (2002). Relieving parentified children's burdens in families with insecure attachment patterns. *Family Process, 41,* 375–388.

Caldwell, B.M., & Bradley, R.H. (2001). *HOME inventory and administration manual* (3rd ed.). Little Rock: University of Arkansas for Medical Sciences and University of Arkansas at Little Rock.

Carlson, V.J., & Harwood, R.L. (1999). Understanding and negotiating cultural difference concerning early developmental competence. *Zero to Three, 20,* 19–24.

Castillo, R.J. (1997). *Culture & mental illness: A client-centered approach.* Pacific Grove, CA: Brooks/Cole.

Caton, C.L.M., Cournos, F., Felix, A., & Wyatt, R.J. (1998). Childhood experiences and current adjustment of offspring of indigent patients with schizophrenia. *Psychiatric Services, 49,* 86–90.

Chandra, P.S., Venkatasubramanian, G., & Thomas, T. (2002). Infanticidal ideas and infanticidal behavior in Indian women with severe postpartum psychiatric disorders. *Journal of Nervous and Mental Disease, 190,* 457–461.

Chaudron, L.H. (2003). Postpartum depression: What pediatricians need to know. *Pediatrics in Review, 14,* 156–161.

Chernomas, W.M., Clarke, D.E., & Chisholm, F.A. (2000). Perspectives of women living with schizophrenia. *Psychiatric Services, 51,* 1517–1521.

Cicchetti, D., & Lynch, M. (1993). Toward an ecological/transactional model of community violence and child maltreatment: Consequences for children's development. *Psychiatry, 56,* 96–118.

Cicchetti, D., Rogosch, F.A., & Toth, S.L. (1998). Maternal depressive disorder and contextual risk: Contributions to the development of attachment insecurity and behavior problems in toddlerhood. *Development and Psychopathology, 10,* 283–300.

Cicchetti, D., & Toth, S. (1995). A developmental psychopathology perspective on child abuse and neglect. *Journal of the American Academy of Child and Adolescent Psychiatry, 34,* 541–565.

Clyman, R.B., Harden, B.J., & Little, C. (2002). Assessment, intervention, and research with infants in out-of-home placement. *Infant Mental Health Journal, 23,* 435–453.

Cohen, L.S., Sichel, D.A., Robertson, L.M., Heckscher, E., & Rosenbaum, J.F. (1995). Postpartum prophylaxis for women with bipolar disorder. *The American Journal of Psychiatry, 152,* 1641–1645.

Cohler, B.F., Stott, F.M., & Musick, J.S. (1996). Distressed parents and their young children: Interventions for families at risk. In M. Göpfert, J. Webster, & M.V. Seeman (Eds.), *Parental psychiatric disorder: Distressed parents and their families* (pp. 107–134). New York: Cambridge University Press.

Cohn, J.F., Campbell, S.B., Matias, R., & Hopkins, J. (1990). Face-to-face interactions of postpartum depressed and nondepressed mother–infant pairs at 2 months. *Developmental Psychology, 26,* 15–23.

Coohey, C. (1996). Child maltreatment: Testing the social isolation hypothesis. *Child Abuse and Neglect: The International Journal, 20,* 241–254.

Corcoran, J. (2000). *Evidence-based social work practice with families: A lifespan approach.* New York: Springer Publishing Company.

Coverdale, J.H., & Aruffo, J.F. (1989). Family planning needs of female chronic psychiatric outpatients. *The American Journal of Psychiatry, 146,* 1489–1491.

Crittenden, P.M. (1982). Abusing, neglecting, problematic, and adequate dyads: Differentiating by patterns of interaction. *Merrill-Palmer Quarterly, 27,* 1–18.

Crittenden, P.M. (1985). Social networks, quality of child rearing and child development. *Child Development, 56,* 1299–1313.

Crittenden, P.M. (1988). Relationships at risk. In J. Belsky & T. Nezworski (Eds.), *Clinical implications of attachment* (pp. 136–174). Hillsdale, NJ: Lawrence Erlbaum Associates.

Crittenden, P.M. (1996). Research on maltreating families: Implications for intervention. In J. Briere, L. Berliner, J.A. Bulkley, C. Jenny, & T. Reid (Eds.), *The APSAC handbook on child maltreatment* (pp. 158–174). Thousand Oaks, CA: Sage Publications.

Crittenden, P.M. (2001, May). *Care-index, coding manual.* Miami, FL: Family Relations Institute.

Crittenden, P.M., & Morrison, A.K. (1988). An early parental indicator of potential maltreatment. *Pediatric Nursing, 14,* 415–417.

Daro, D. (1996). Preventing child abuse and neglect. In J. Briere, L. Berliner, J.A. Bulkley, C. Jenny, & T. Reid (Eds.), *The APSAC handbook on child maltreatment* (pp. 343–358). Thousand Oaks, CA: Sage Publications.

David, A. (1990). Insight and psychosis. *British Journal of Psychiatry, 156,* 798–808.

Davies, A., McIvor, R., & Kumar, R. (1995). Impact of childbirth on a series of schizophrenic mothers: Possible influence of estrogen on schizophrenia. *Schizophrenia Research, 16,* 25–31.

DeMulder, E.K., & Radke-Yarrow, M. (1991). Attachment with affectively ill and well mothers: Concurrent behavioral correlates. *Development and Psychopathology, 3,* 227–242.

DeMulder, E.K., Tarulla, L.B., Klimes-Dougan, B., Free, K., & Radke-Yarrow, M. (1995). Personality disorders of affectively ill mothers: Links to maternal behavior. *Journal of Personality Disorders, 9,* 199–212.

Diaz-Caneja, A., & Johnson, S. (2004). The views and experiences of severely mentally ill mothers: A qualitative study. *Social Psychiatry and Psychiatric Epidemiology, 39,* 472–482.

Dinwiddie, S., & Bucholz, K. (1993). Psychiatric diagnoses of self-reported child abusers. *Child Abuse and Neglect: The International Journal, 17,* 465–476.

Dolan, M., & Doyle, M. (2000). Violence risk prediction: Clinical and actuarial measures and the role of the psychopathy checklist. *British Journal of Psychiatry, 177,* 303–311.

Eastwood, J., Spielvogel, A., & Wile, J. (1990). Countertransference risks when women treat women. *Clinical Social Work Journal, 18,* 273–280.

Edleson, J.L. (1999). The overlap between child maltreatment and woman battering. *Violence Against Women, 5,* 134–154.

Egeland, B., Bosquet, M., & Chung, A.L. (2002). Continuities and discontinuities in the intergenerational transmission of child maltreatment: Implications for breaking the cycle of abuse. In K.D. Browne, H. Hanks, P. Stratton, & C.E. Hamilton (Eds.), *Early prediction and prevention of child abuse: A handbook* (pp. 217–232). Chichester, England: Wiley.

Egeland, B., Carlson, E., & Sroufe, L.A. (1993). Resilience as process. *Development and Psychopathology, 5,* 517–528.

Egeland, B., & Erickson, M.F. (1987). Psychologically unavailable caregiving. In M. Brassard, R. Germain, & S. Hart (Eds.), *Psychological maltreatment of children and youth* (pp. 110–120). New York: Pergamon Press.

Fendrich, M., Warner, V., & Weissman, M.M. (1990). Family risk factors, parental depression, and psychopathology in offspring. *Developmental Psychology, 26,* 40–50.

Fink, L.A., Bernstein, D., Handelsman, L., Foote, J., & Lovejoy, M. (1995). Initial validity and reliability of the childhood trauma interview: A new multidimensional measure of a childhood interpersonal trauma. *The American Journal of Psychiatry, 152,* 1329–1335.

Finnerty, M., Levin, Z., & Miller, L.J. (1996). Acute manic episodes in pregnancy (clinical conference). *American Journal of Psychiatry, 153,* 261–263.

Fitzpatrick, G. (1995). Assessing treatability. In P. Reder & C. Lucey (Eds.), *Assessment of parenting: Psychiatric and psychological contributions* (pp. 102–117). London: Routledge.

Fitzpatrick, G., Reder, P., & Lucey, C. (1995). The child's perspective. In P. Reder & C. Lucey (Eds.), *Assessment of parenting: Psychiatric and psychological contributions* (pp. 56–72). London: Routledge.

Flynn, A., Matthews, H., & Hollins, S. (2002). Validity of the diagnosis of personality disorder in adults with learning disability and severe behavior problems. *British Journal of Psychiatry, 180,* 543–546.

Foley, D.L., Maes, H.H., Silberg, J.L., Pickles, A., Simonoff, E., Hewitt, J.K., et al. (2001). Parental concordance and comorbidity for psychiatric disorder and associated risks for current psychiatric symptoms and disorders in a community sample of juvenile twins. *Journal of Child Psychology and Psychiatry and Applied Disciplines, 42,* 381–394.

Folman, R.D. (1998). "I was tooken": How children experience removal from their parents preliminary to placement into foster care. *Adoption Quarterly, 2,* 7–35.

Forehand, R., & McMahon, R. (1981). *Helping the noncompliant child: A clinician's guide to parent training.* New York: Guilford Press.

Forehand, R., Wells, K., & Griest, D. (1980). An examination of the social validity of a parent-training program. *Behavior Therapy, 11,* 488–502.

Fox, L. (1999). Personal accounts: Missing out on motherhood. *Psychiatric Services, 50,* 193–194.

Fraiberg, S.H., Adelson, E., & Shapiro, V. (1987). Ghosts in the nursery: A psychoanalytic approach to the problems of impaired infant–mother relationships. In L. Fraiberg (Ed.), *Selected writings of Selma Fraiberg (pp. 100–136).* Columbus: Ohio State University Press.

Gabbard, G.O. (2000). *Psychodynamic psychiatry in clinical practice: The* DSM-IV *edition* (3rd ed.). Washington, DC: American Psychiatric Press.

Gambrill, E. (2005). *Critical thinking in clinical practice: Improving the quality of judgments and decisions* (2nd ed.). Hoboken, NJ: John Wiley & Sons.

Gambrill, E. (2006). Evidence-based practice and policy: Choices ahead. *Research on Social Work Practice, 16,* 338–357.

Garcia, M.M., Shaw, D.S., Winslow, E.B., & Yaggi, K.E. (2000). Destructive sibling conflict and the development of conduct problems in young boys. *Developmental Psychology, 36,* 44–53.

Gaudin, J.M., Polansky, N.A., & Kilpatrick, A.C. (1992). The child well-being scales: A field trial. *Child Welfare, 71,* 319–328.

Gaudin, J.M., Polansky, N.A., Kilpatrick, A.C., & Shilton, P. (1993). Loneliness, depression, stress, and social supports in neglectful families. *American Journal of Orthopsychiatry, 63,* 597–605.

George, C., & Main, M. (1984). *Attachment interview for adults.* Unpublished manuscript, University of California at Berkeley.

George, C., & Solomon, J. (1989). Internal working models of parenting and security of attachment at age six. *Infant Mental Health Journal, 10,* 222–237.

George, C., & Solomon, J. (1996). Representational models of relationships: Links between caregiving and attachment. *Infant Mental Health Journal, 17,* 198–216.

Germain, C.B., & Bloom, M. (1999). *Human behavior in the social environment: An ecological view* (2nd ed.). New York: Columbia University Press.

Ghaemi, S.N. (1999). Performative statements and the will: Mechanisms of psychotherapeutic change. *American Journal of Psychotherapy, 53,* 483–494.

Gil, D.G. (1987). Maltreatment as a function of the structure of social systems. In M.R. Brassard, R. Germain, & S.N. Hart (Eds.), *Psychological maltreatment of children and youth* (pp. 159–170). New York: Pergamon Press.

Gilkerson, L., & Shahmoon-Shanok, R. (2000). Relationships for growth: Cultivating reflective practice in infant, toddler, and preschool programs. In J.D. Osofsky & H.E. Fitzgerald (Eds.), *WAIMH handbook of infant mental health: Vol. 2. Early intervention, evaluation and assessment* (pp. 3–32). New York: John Wiley & Sons.

Goldstein, J., Solnit, A.J., Goldstein, S., & Freud, A. (1998). *The best interests of the child: The least detrimental alternative.* New York: Free Press.

Goodman, S.H., & Emory, E.K. (1992). Perinatal complications in births to low socioeconomic status schizophrenic and depressed women. *Journal of Abnormal Psychology, 101,* 225–229.

Goodman, S.H., & Gotlib, I.H. (1999). Risk for psychopathology in the children of depressed mothers: A developmental model for understanding mechanisms of transmission. *Psychological Review, 106,* 458–490.

Göpfert, M., Webster, J., & Nelki, J. (2004a). The construction of parenting and its context. In M. Göpfert, J. Webster, & M.V. Seeman (Eds.), *Parental Psychiatric disorder: Distressed parents and their families* (2nd ed., pp. 62–86, 93–111). Cambridge, England: Cambridge University Press.

Göpfert, M., Webster, J., & Nelki, J. (2004b). Formulation and assessment of parenting. In M. Göpfert, J. Webster, M.V. Seeman (Eds.), *Parental psychiatric disorder: Distressed parents and their families,* (2nd ed.; pp. 93–111). Cambridge, England: Cambridge University Press.

Göpfert, M., Webster, J., & Seeman, M.V. (Eds.). (2004). *Parental psychiatric disorder: Distressed parents and their families* (2nd ed.). Cambridge, England: Cambridge University Press.

Goldstein, A.P., Keller, H., & Erne, D. (1985). *Changing the abusive parent.* Champaign, IL: Research Press.

Greene, B.F., Tertinger, D., Sievert, D., Montes, A., Kilili, S., Dunne, R., et al. (n.d.). *An observer training manual for project 12-ways staff: The home accident prevention inventory.* Carbondale, IL: Project 12-ways.

Greif, G.L., & Drechsler, M. (1993). Common issues for parents in a methadone maintenance group. *Journal of Substance Abuse Treatment, 10,* 339–343.

Grisso, T. (2002). *Evaluating competencies: Forensic assessments and instruments* (2nd ed.). New York: Springer.

Grisso, T., & Appelbaum, P.S. (1992). Is it unethical to offer predictions of future violence? *Law and Human Behavior, 16,* 621–633.

Grunbaum, L., & Gammeltoft, M. (1993).Young children of schizophrenic mothers: Difficulties of intervention. *American Journal of Orthopsychiatry, 63,* 16–27.

Haight, W.L., Black, J.E., Workman, C., & Tata, L. (2001). Parent–child interactions during foster care visits: Implications for practice. *Social Work, 46,* 325–338.

Haight, W., & Miller, P. (1993). *Pretending at home: Early development in a sociocultural context.* Albany: State University of New York Press.

Hall, A. (2004). Parental psychiatric disorder and the developing child. In M. Göpfert, J. Webster, & M.V. Seeman (Eds.), *Parental psychiatric disorder: Distressed parents and their families* (2nd ed., pp. 22–49). Cambridge, England: Cambridge University Press.

Hamilton, J.A., & Sichel, D.A. (1992). Prophylactic measures. In J.A. Hamilton & P.N. Harberger (Eds.), *Postpartum psychiatric illness: A picture puzzle* (pp. 219–254). Philadelphia: University of Pennsylvania Press.

Hammen, C., & Brennan, P.A. (2003). Severity, chronicity, and timing of maternal depression and risk for adolescent offspring diagnoses in a community sample. *Archives of General Psychiatry, 60,* 253–258.

Hans, S.L. (1999). Demographic and psychosocial characteristics of substance abusing pregnant women. *Clinics in Perinatology, 26,* 55–74.

Hans, S.L. (2004). When mothers abuse drugs. In M. Göpfert, J. Webster, & M.V. Seeman (Eds.), *Parental psychiatric disorder: Distressed parents and their families* (2nd ed., pp. 203–216). Cambridge, England: Cambridge University Press.

Hansburg, H.G. (1972). *Adolescent separation anxiety: A method for the study of adolescent separation problems.* Springfield, IL: Charles C. Thomas.

Harter, S. (1985). *Manual for the self-perception profile for children.* Denver, CO: University of Denver.

Harter, S. (1988). *Manual for the self-perception profile for adolescents.* Denver, CO: University of Denver.

Hartman, A. (1995). Diagrammatic assessment of family relationships. *Families in Society, 76,* 111–122.

Hatfield, B., Webster, J., & Mohamad, U. (1997). Psychiatric emergencies: Assessing parents of dependent children. *Psychiatric Bulletin, 21,* 19–22.

Heinicke, C.M., & Westheimer, I. (1965). *Brief separations.* New York: International Universities Press.

Herbert, M., & Harper-Dorton, K. (2002). *Working with children, adolescents, and their families* (3rd ed.). Chicago: Lyceum Books.

Herman, S.P. (1997). Practice parameters for the American Academy of Child and Adolescent Psychiatry: Child custody evaluation. *Journal of the American Academy of Child and Adolescent Psychiatry: Practice Parameters, 36*(Suppl. 10), 57S–68S.

Heron, J., O'Connor, T.G., Evans, J., Golding, J., Glover, V., & the ALSPAC Study Team. (2004). The course of anxiety and depression through pregnancy and the postpartum in a community sample. *Journal of Affective Disorders, 80,* 65–73.

Hesse, E. (1999). The adult attachment interview: Historical and current perspectives. In J. Cassidy & P.R. Shaver (Eds.), *Handbook of attachment: Theory, research and clinical application* (pp. 395–433). New York: Guilford Press.

Hibbs, E.D., Hamburger, S.D., Kruesi, M.J., & Lenane, M. (1993). Factors affecting expressed emotion in parents of ill and normal children. *American Journal of Orthopsychiatry, 63,* 103–112.

Hibbs, E.D., Hamburger, S.D., Lenane, M., Rapoport, J.L., Kruesi, M.J., Keysor, C.S., et al. (1991). Determinants of expressed emotion in families of disturbed and normal children. *Journal of Child Psychology and Psychiatry and Applied Disciplines, 32,* 757–770.

Hill, J., Fonagy, P., Safier, E., & Sargent, J. (2003). The ecology of attachment in the family. *Family Process, 42,* 205–221.

Hill, N.E., & Bush, K.R. (2001, November). Relationships between parenting environment and children's mental health among African American and European American mothers and children. *Journal of Marriage and Family, 63,* 954–966.

Hipwell, A.E., Goossens, F.A., Melhuish, E.C., & Kumar, R. (2000). Severe maternal psychopathology and infant–mother attachment. *Development and Psychopathology, 12,* 157–175.

Hodges, J., Steele, S., Hillman, S., Henderson, K., & Kaniuk, J. (2003). Changes in attachment representations over the first year of adoptive placement: Narratives of maltreated children. *Clinical Child Psychology and Psychiatry, 8,* 351–367.

Holley, T.E., & Holley, J. (1997). *My mother's keeper: A daughter's memoir of growing up in the shadow of schizophrenia.* New York: William Morrow.

Hynan, D.J. (2003). Parent–child observations in custody evaluations. *Family Court Review, 41,* 214–223.

Illinois Department of Children and Family Services, Office of the Inspector General. (1999). *Home safety checklist.* Chicago: Author.

Jacobsen, T. (2004). Mentally ill mothers in the parenting role: Clinical management and treatment. In M. Göpfert, J. Webster, & M.V. Seeman (Eds.), *Parental psychiatric disorder: Distressed parents and their families* (2nd ed., p. 113). England: Cambridge University Press.

Jacobsen, T., Edelstein, W., & Hofmann, V. (1994). A longitudinal study of the relation between representations of attachment in childhood and cognitive functioning in childhood and adolescence. *Developmental Psychology, 30,* 112–124.

Jacobsen, T., Hibbs, E., & Ziegenhain, U. (2000). Maternal expressed emotion related to attachment disorganization in early childhood: A preliminary report. *Journal of Child Psychology and Psychiatry and Applied Disciplines, 41,* 899–906.

Jacobsen, T., Levy-Chung, A., & Kim, J. (2002). Intervening with young children in foster care: Using countertransference reactions to facilitate the therapeutic process. *Zero to Three, 25*(3), 57–60.

Jacobsen, T., & Miller, L.J. (1998a). Compulsive compliance in a young maltreated child. *Journal of the American Academy of Child and Adolescent Psychiatry, 37,* 462–463.

Jacobsen, T., & Miller, L.J. (1998b). Focus on women: Mentally ill mothers who have killed: Three cases addressing the issue of future parenting capability. *Psychiatric Services, 49,* 650–657.

Jacobsen, T., & Miller, L.J. (1999). The caregiving contexts of young children who have been removed from the care of a mentally ill mother: Relations to mother–child attachment quality. In J. Solomon & C. George (Eds.), *Attachment disorganization* (pp. 347–378). New York: Guilford Press.

Jacobsen, T., Miller, L.J., & Kirkwood, K. (1997). Assessing parenting competency in individuals with severe mental illness: A comprehensive service. *Journal of Mental Health Administration, 24,* 189–199.

Jenkins, E.J., & Bell, C.C. (1997). Exposure and response to community violence among children and adolescents. In J. Osofsky (Ed.), *Children in a violent society* (pp. 9–31). New York: Guilford Press.

Jofesson, A., Berg, G., Nordin, C., & Sydsjö, G. (2001). Prevalence of depressive symptoms in late pregnancy and postpartum. *Acta Obstetricia et Gynecologica Scandinavica, 80,* 251–255.

Jolowicz, A.R. (1969). The hidden parent. In *Source Book of Teaching Materials on the Welfare of Children* (pp. 105–110). New York: Council of Social Work Education.

Jordan, C., & Franklin, C. (2003). *Clinical assessment for social workers: Quantitative and qualitative methods* (2nd ed.). Chicago: Lyceum Books.

Jurkovic, G.H. (1997). *Lost childhoods: The plight of the parentified child.* New York: Brunner/ Mazel.

Kaltenbach, K. & Finnegan, L.P. (1987). Perinatal and developmental outcome of infants exposed to methadone in-utero. *Neurotoxicology and Teratology, 9,* 311–313.

Kemp, S.P., Whittaker, J.K., & Tracy, E.M. (1997). *Person-environment practice: The social ecology of interpersonal helping.* Hawthorne, NY: Aldine de Gruyter.

Kempe, R.S., & Kempe, H. (1978). *Child abuse.* Cambridge, MA: Harvard University Press.

Kitzmann, K.M., Gaylord, N.K., Holt, A.R., & Kenny, E.D. (2003). Child witnesses to domestic violence: A meta-analytic review. *Journal of Consulting and Clinical Psychology, 71,* 339–352.

Klee, H. (1998). Drug-using parents: Analysing the stereotypes. *The International Journal of Drug Policy, 9,* 437–448.

Kluft, R.P. (1987). The parental fitness of mothers with multiple personality disorder: A preliminary study. *Child Abuse and Neglect: The International Journal, 11,* 273–280.

Knutson, J.F., & Bower, M.E. (1994). Physically abusive parenting as an escalated aggressive response. In M. Potegal & J.F. Knutson (Eds.), *The dynamics of aggression: Biological and social processes in dyads and groups* (pp. 195–225). Hillsdale, NJ: Lawrence Erlbaum Associates.

Kochanska, G., Kuczynski, L., Radke-Yarrow, M., & Darby-Welsh, J.D. (1987). Resolutions of control episodes between well and affectively ill mothers and their young children. *Journal of Abnormal Child Psychology, 15,* 441–456.

Kovacs, M. (1985). The Children's Depression Inventory (CDI). *Psychopharmacology Bulletin, 21,* 995–998.

Kroll, B. (2004). Living with an elephant: Growing up with parental substance misuse. *Child & Family Social Work, 9,* 129–140.

Kumar, R., Marks, M., Platz, C., & Yoshida, K. (1995). Clinical survey of a psychiatric mother and baby unit: Characteristics of 100 consecutive admissions. *Journal of Affective Disorders, 33,* 11–22.

Leventhal, J.M., Forsyth, B.W.C., Qi, K., Johnson, L., Schroeder, C., & Votto, N. (1997). Maltreatment of children born to mothers who used cocaine during pregnancy: A population-based study. *Pediatrics, 100,* 2–7.

Lieberman, A.F. (1989). What is culturally sensitive intervention? *Early Child Development and Care, 50,* 197–204.

Lieberman, A.F. (1990). Culturally sensitive intervention with children and families. *Child & Adolescent Social Work Journal, 17,* 101–120.

Lieberman, A.F. (1993). *The emotional life of the toddler.* New York: Free Press.

Lieberman, A.F., Compton, N.C., Van Horn, P., Ghosh Ippen, C. (2003). *Losing a parent to death in the early years: Guidelines for the treatment of traumatic bereavement in infancy and early childhood.* Washington, DC: ZERO TO THREE.

Lieberman, A.F., Padron, E., Van Horn, P., & Harris, W.E. (2005). Angels in the nursery: The intergenerational transmission of benevolent parental influences. *Infant Mental Health Journal, 26,* 504–520.

Lieberman, A.F., & Van Horn, P. (2005). *Don't hit my mommy! A manual for child–parent psychotherapy with young witnesses of family violence.* Washington, DC: ZERO TO THREE.

Lincoln, Y.S., & Guba, E.G. (1985). *Naturalistic inquiry.* Beverly Hills, CA: Sage Publications.

Link, B.G., & Cullen, F.T. (1986). Contact with the mentally ill and perceptions of how dangerous they are. *Journal of Health and Social Behavior, 27,* 289–302.

Luthar, S.S., & Walsh, K. (1995). Treatment needs of drug-addicted mothers: Integrated parenting psychotherapy interventions. *Journal of Substance Abuse Treatment, 12,* 341–348.

Lynch, M.A., & Roberts, J. (1977). Predicting child abuse: Signs of bonding failure in the maternity hospital. *British Medical Journal, 1,* 624–626.

Lyons-Ruth, K., & Jacobvitz, D. (1999). Attachment disorganization: Unresolved loss, relational violence, and lapses in behavioral and attentional strategies. In J. Cassidy & P.R. Shaver (Eds.), *Handbook of attachment theory and research* (pp. 520–544). New York: Guilford Press.

Lyons-Ruth, K., Wolfe, R., & Lyubchik, A. (2000). Depression and the parenting of young children: Making the case for early preventive mental health services. *Harvard Review of Psychiatry, 8,* 148–153.

Lyons-Ruth, K., Yellin, C., Melnick, S., & Atwood, G. (2005). Expanding the concept of unresolved mental states: Hostile/helpless states of mind on the adult attachment interview are associated with disrupted mother–infant communication and infant disorganization. *Development and Psychopathology, 17,* 1–23.

Lysaker, P., Bell, M., Milstein, R., Bryson, G., & Beam-Goulet, J. (1994). Insight and psychological treatment compliance in schizophrenia. *Psychiatry, 57,* 307–315.

MacQueen, G.M., Young, L.T., & Joffe, R.T. (2001). A review of psychosocial outcome in patients with bipolar disorder. *Acta Psychiatrica Scandinavica, 103,* 163–170.

Magana, A.B., Goldstein, M.J., Karno, M., Miklowitz, D.J., Jenkins, J., & Falloon, I.R. (1986). A brief method for assessing expressed emotion in relatives of psychiatric patients. *Psychiatry Research, 17,* 203–212.

Magana-Amato, A. (1993, May). *Manual for coding expressed emotion from the five minute speech sample.* Unpublished manuscript, University of California at Los Angeles.

Magura, S., & Moses, B.S. (1986). *Outcome measures for child welfare services: Theory and applications.* Washington, DC: Child Welfare League of America.

Marsh, D.T. (1998). *Serious mental illness and the family: The practitioner's guide.* Somerset, NJ: John Wiley & Sons.

Martins, C., & Gaffan, E.A. (2000). Effects of early maternal depression on patterns of infant–mother attachment: A meta-analytic investigation. *Journal of Child Psychology and Psychiatry and Applied Disciplines, 41,* 737–746.

Mattaini, M.A. (1993). *More than a thousand words: Graphics for clinical practice.* Washington, DC: NASW Press.

Mattaini, M.A., & Meyer, C.H. (2002). The ecosystems perspective: Implications for practice. In M.A. Mattaini, C.T. Lowery, & C.H. Meyer (Eds.), *Foundations of social work practice* (pp. 3–24). Washington, DC: NASW Press.

McEvoy, J.P., Appelbaum, P.S., Apperson, L.J., Geller, J.L., & Freter, S. (1989). Why must some schizophrenic patients be involuntarily committed? The role of insight. *Comprehensive Psychiatry, 30,* 13–17.

McGoldrick, M., Gerson, R., & Shellenberger, S. (1999). *Genograms: Assessment and intervention.* New York: W.W. Norton & Company.

McMahon, R.J., & Forehand, R.L. (1984). Parent training for the non-compliant child: Treatment outcome, generalization and adjunctive therapy procedures. In R.F. Dangel & R.A. Polster (Eds.), *Parent training: Foundations of research and practice* (pp. 298–328). New York: Guilford Press.

McNeil, T.F., Persson-Blennow, I., Binett, B., Harty, B., & Karyd, U.B. (1988). A prospective study of post-partum psychoses in a high-risk group: 7. Relation to later offspring characteristics. *Acta Psychiatrica Scandinavica, 78,* 613–617.

Meisels, S.J. (2001). Fusing assessment and intervention: Changing parents' and providers' views of young children. *Zero to Three, 21*(4), 4–10.

Merikangas, K.R., Dierker, L.C., & Szatmari, P. (1998). Psychopathology among offspring of parents with substance abuse and/or anxiety disorders: A high-risk study. *The Journal of Psychology and Psychiatry and Allied Disciplines, 39,* 711–720.

Miller, A. (1983). *The drama of the gifted child and the search for the true self.* London: Faber and Faber.

Miller, L.J. (1997). Sexuality, reproduction, and family planning in women with schizophrenia. *Schizophrenia Bulletin, 23,* 623–635.

Miller, L.J. (2002). Postpartum depression. *JAMA: The Journal of the American Medical Association, 287,* 762–765.

Miller, L.J., & Finnerty, M. (1996). Sexuality, pregnancy, and childrearing among women with schizophrenia-spectrum disorders. *Psychiatric Services, 47,* 502–506.

Miller, L.J., Jacobsen, T., Jones, V., Reyes, J., Kim, J., & Garcia, M. (1998). *Parenting assessment team training manual.* Chicago: University of Illinois at Chicago.

Millis, J.B., & Kornblith, P.R. (1992). Fragile beginnings: Identification and treatment of postpartum disorders. *Health & Social Work, 17,* 192–199.

Milner, J.S. (1980). *The child abuse potential inventory: Manual.* Webster, NC: Psytec.

Monahan, J. (1992). Mental disorder and violent behavior: Perceptions and evidence. *American Psychologist, 47*(4), 511–521.

Monahan, J. (1996). Violence prediction: The past twenty and next twenty years. *Criminal Justice and Behavior, 23,* 107–120.

Monahan, J., Steadman, H.J., Robbins, P.C., Silver, E., Appelbaum, P.S., Grisso, T., et al. (2000). Developing a clinically useful actuarial tool for assessing violence risk. *British Journal of Psychiatry, 176,* 312–319.

Mowbray, C.T., Oyserman, D., Zemencuk, J.K., & Ross, S.R. (1995). Motherhood for women with serious mental illness: Pregnancy, childbirth, and the postpartum period. *American Journal of Orthopsychiatry, 65,* 21–38.

Mullick, M., Miller, L.J., & Jacobsen, T. (2001). Insight into mental illness and child maltreatment risk in mothers with major psychiatric disorders. *Psychiatric Services, 52,* 488–492.

Murphy, P. (1996, June/July). Diverting abuse cases from juvenile court: Has the due process revolution gone too far? *Chicago Bar Association Record,* 30–34.

Murray, L., Sinclair, D., Cooper, P., Ducournau, P., Turner, P., & Stein, A. (1999). The socio-emotional development of 5-year-old children of postnatally depressed mothers. *The Journal of Child Psychology and Psychiatry and Applied Disciplines, 40,* 1259–1272.

National Institute of Child Health and Human Development (n.d.). SIDS: "Back to sleep" campaign. Retrieved January 24, 2004, from http://www.nichd.nih.gov/sids/sids.cfm

Nicholson, J., & Biebel, K. (2002). Commentary on "Community mental health care for women with severe mental illness who are parents"—The tragedy of missed opportunities: What providers can do. *Community Mental Health Journal, 38,* 167–172.

Nicholson, J., Biebel, K., Hinden, B., Henry, A., & Stier, L. (2001). *Critical issues for parents with mental illness and their families* (KEN01–0109). Rockville, MD: Center for Mental Health Services, Substance Abuse and Mental Health Services Administration.

Nicholson, J., & Blanch, A. (1994). Rehabilitation for parenting roles for people with serious mental illness. *Psychosocial Rehabilitation Journal, 18,* 109–119.

Nicholson, J., Geller, J.L., Fisher, W.H., & Dion, G.L. (1993). State policies and programs that address the needs of mentally ill mothers in the public sector. *Hospital and Community Psychiatry, 44,* 484–489.

Nicholson, J., Nason, M.W., Calebresi, A.O., & Yando, R. (1999). Fathers with severe mental illness: Characteristics and comparisons. *American Journal of Orthopsychiatry, 69,* 134–141.

Nicholson, J., Sweeney, E.M., & Geller, J.L. (1998a). Focus on women: Mothers with mental illness: I. The competing demands of parenting and living with mental illness. *Psychiatric Services, 49,* 635–642.

Nicholson, J., Sweeney, E.M., & Geller, J.L. (1998b). Focus on women: Mothers with mental illness: II. Family relationships and the context of parenting. *Psychiatric Services, 49,* 643–649.

Norton, K., & Dolan, B. (1996). Personality disorder and parenting. In M. Göpfert, J. Webster, & M.V. Seeman (Eds.), *Parental psychiatric disorder: Distressed parents and their families* (pp. 219–323). Cambridge, England: Cambridge University Press.

Oates, M. (1997). Patients as parents: The risk to children. *British Journal of Psychiatry, 170*(Suppl. 32), 22–27.

O'Connor, T.G., Hawkins, N., Dunn, J., Thorpe, K., & Golding, J. (1998). Family type and depression in pregnancy: Factors mediating risk in a community sample. *Journal of Marriage and Family, 60,* 757–770.

O'Hara, M.W. (1986). Social support, life events, and depression during pregnancy and the puerperium. *Archives of General Psychiatry, 43,* 569–573.

O'Hara, M.W., Neunaber, D.J., & Zekoski, E.M. (1984). Prospective study of postpartum depression: Prevalence, course and predictive factors. *Journal of Abnormal Psychology, 93,* 158–171.

O'Hara, M.W., Zekoski, E.M., Philipps, L.H., & Wright, E.J. (1990). Controlled prospective study of postpartum mood disorders: Comparison of childbearing and nonchildbearing women. *Journal of Abnormal Psychology, 99,* 3–15.

Oppenheim, D., Emde, R.N., & Warren, S. (1997). Emotion regulation in mother–child narrative co-construction: Associations with children's narratives and adaptation. *Development and Psychopathology, 33,* 284–294.

Ostler, T., & Haight, W.L. (n.d.). Viewing young foster children's responses to visits through the lens of maternal containment: Implications for attachment disorganization. In J. Solomon & C. George (Eds.), *Attachment disorganization* (2nd ed.). New York: Guilford Press.

Ostler, T., Haight, W., Black, J., Choi, G.Y., Kingery, L., & Sheridan, K. (2007). Mental health outcomes and perspectives of rural children reared by parents who abuse methamphetamine. *Journal of the American Academy of Child and Adolescent Psychiatry, 46,* 500–507.

Oyserman, D., Mowbray, C.T., Allen-Meares, P., & Firminger, K. (2000). Parenting among mothers with a serious mental illness. *American Journal of Orthopsychiatry, 70,* 296–315.

Oyserman, D., Mowbray, C.T., & Zemencuk, J.K. (1994). Resources and supports for mothers with severe mental illness. *Health & Social Work, 19,* 132–142.

Parker, G.R., Cowen, W.L., Work, W.C., & Wyman, P.A. (1990). Test correlates of stress resilience among urban school children. *The Journal of Primary Prevention, 11,* 19–35.

Patterson, G. (1982). *Coercive family processes.* Eugene, OR: Castalia Publications.

Patterson, G.R., Reid, J.B., Jones, R.R., & Conger, R.E. (1975). *A social learning approach to family intervention: Families with aggressive children* (Vol. 1). Eugene, OR: Castalia Publications.

Pawl, J.H., & St. John, M. (1998). *How you are is as important as what you do . . . in making a positive difference for infants, toddlers, and their families.* Washington, DC: ZERO TO THREE.

Persson-Blennow, I., Binett, T.F., & McNeil, T. (1988). Offspring of women with nonorganic psychosis: Antecedents of anxious attachment to the mother at one year of age. *Acta Psychiatrica Scandinavica, 78,* 66–71.

Polansky, N.A. (1986). *Treating loneliness in child protection.* Washington, DC: Child Welfare League of America.

Polansky, N.A., Cabral, R.J., Magura, S., & Phillips, M.H. (1983). Comparative norms for the Childhood Level of Living Scale. *Journal of Social Service Research, 6,* 45–55.

Polansky, N.A., Chalmers, M.A., Buttenweiser, E., & Williams, D. (1978). Assessing adequacy of child caring: An urban scale. *Child Welfare, 47,* 439–449.

Polansky, N.A., Gaudin, J.M., Ammon, P.W., & Davis, I.B. (1985). The psychological ecology of the neglectful mother. *Child Abuse and Neglect: The International Journal, 9,* 265–275.

Radke-Yarrow, M., McCann, K., DeMulder, E., Belmont, B., Martinez, P., & Richardson, D.T. (1995). Attachment in the context of high-risk conditions. *Development and Psychopathology, 7,* 247–265.

Radke-Yarrow, M., Nottelmann, E., Belmont, B., & Welsh, J.D. (1995). Affective interactions of depressed and nondepressed mothers and their children. *Journal of Abnormal Child Psychology, 21,* 683–695.

Ramchandani, P., & Stein, A. (2003). The impact of parental psychiatric disorder on children. *British Medical Journal, 327,* 242–243.

Reder, P., & Lucey, C. (Eds.). (1995a). *Assessment of parenting: Psychiatric and psychological contributions.* London: Routledge.

Reder, P., & Lucey, C. (1995b). Significant issues in the assessment of parenting. In P. Reder & C. Lucey (Eds.), *Assessment of parenting: Psychiatric and psychological contributions* (pp. 3–17). London: Routledge.

Reder, P., McClure, M., & Jolley, A. (2000). *Family matters: Interfaces between child and adult mental health.* London: Routledge.

Reid, J.B. (1978). *A social learning approach to family intervention: Observation in home settings* (Vol. 2). Eugene, OR: Castalia Publications.

Reynolds, W.M. (1992). Introduction to the nature and study of internalizing disorders in children and adolescents. In W.M. Reynolds (Ed.), *Internalizing disorders in children and adolescents* (pp. 1–18). New York: John Wiley & Sons.

Righetti-Veltema, M., Bousquet, A., & Manzano, J. (2003). Impact of postpartum depressive symptoms on mother and her 18-month infant. *European Child & Adolescent Psychiatry, 12,* 75–83.

Ritscher, J.E.B., Coursey, R.D., & Farrell, E.W. (1997). A survey on the lives of women with severe mental illness. *Psychiatric Services, 48,* 1273–1282.

Robertson, J., & Robertson, J. (1982). *Baby in the family.* London: Penguin Books.

Robertson, J., & Robertson, J. (1989). *Separation and the very young.* London: Free Association Books.

Robins, L.N. (1966). *Deviant children grown up: A sociological and psychiatric study of sociopathic personality.* Baltimore: Lippincott Williams and Wilkins.

Rodning, C., Beckwith, L., & Howard, J. (1989). Characteristics of attachment organization and play organization in prenatally drug-exposed toddlers. *Development and Psychopathology, 1,* 277–289.

Ruppert, S., & Bagedahl-Strindlund, M. (2001). Children of parapartum mentally ill mothers: A follow-up study. *Psychopathology, 34,* 174–178.

Rutter, M. (1985). Resilience in the face of adversity: Protective factors and resistance to psychiatric disorder. *British Journal of Psychiatry, 147,* 598–611.

Rutter, M. (1986). Parental mental disorder as a psychiatric risk factor. *Psychological Association Annual Review, 6,* 647–663.

Rutter, M. (1995). Clinical implications of attachment concepts: Retrospect and prospect. *Journal of Child Psychology and Psychiatry and Applied Disciplines, 36,* 549–571.

Rutter, M., Quinton, D., & Liddle, C. (1983). Parenting in two generations: Looking backwards and looking forwards. In N. Madge (Ed.), *Families at risk* (pp. 60–98). London: Heinemann Educational.

Ryle, A., & Kerr, I. (2002). *Introducing cognitive-analytic therapy: Principles and practice.* Chichester, England: John Wiley & Sons.

Sackheim, H.A. (1998). The meaning of insight. In X.F. Amador & A.S. David (Eds.), *Insight and psychosis* (pp. 3–12). New York: Oxford University Press.

Sagi, A., van IJzendoorn, M.H., Scharf, M., Koren–Karie, N., Joels, T., & Mayseless, O. (1994). Stability and discriminant validity of the Adult Attachment Interview: A psychometric study in young Israeli adults. *Developmental Psychology, 30,* 771–777.

Sameroff, A.J., Seifer, R., & Zax, M. (1982). Early development of children at risk for emotional disorder. *Monographs of the Society for Research in Child Development, 47(Serial No. 199),* 1–82.

Schachnow, J., Clarkin, J., DiPalma, C.S., Thurston, F., Hull, J., & Shearin, E. (1997). Parental psychopathology and borderline personality disorder. *Psychiatry, 60,* 171–181.

Schmitt, B.D. (1987). Seven deadly sins of childhood: Advising parents about difficult developmental phases. *Child Abuse & Neglect: The International Journal, 11,* 421–432.

Schuler, M.E., Nair, P., Black, M.M., & Kettinger, L. (2000). Mother–infant interaction: Effects of a home intervention and ongoing maternal drug use. *Journal of Child Clinical Psychology, 29,* 424–431.

Schwartz, C.E., Dorer, D.J., Beardslee, W.R., Lavori, P.W., & Keller, M.B. (1990). Maternal expressed emotion and parental affective disorder: Risk for childhood depressive disorder, substance abuse, or conduct disorder. *Journal of Psychiatric Research, 24,* 231–250.

Seeman, M.V. (2006). Schizophrenia during pregnancy and the postpartum period. In V. Hendrick (Ed.), *Psychiatric disorders in pregnancy and the postpartum: Principles and treatment* (pp. 139–152). Totowa, NJ: Humana Press.

Seeman, M.V., & Göpfert, M. (2004). Parenthood and adult mental health. In M. Göpfert, J. Webster, & M.V. Seeman (Eds.), *Parental psychiatric disorder: Distressed parents and their families* (2nd ed., pp. 8–21). Cambridge, UK: Cambridge University Press.

Shahmoon-Shanok, R., Gilkerson, L., Eggbeer, L., & Fenichel, E. (1995). *Reflective supervision: A relationship for learning.* Washington, DC: ZERO TO THREE.

Shakel, J.A. (1987). Emotional neglect and stimulus deprivation. In M. Brassard, R. Germain, & S. Hart (Eds.), *Psychological maltreatment of children and youth* (pp. 100–109). New York: Pergamon Press.

Shonkoff, J.P. (2000). Science, policy, and practice: Three cultures in search of a shared mission. *Child Development, 71,* 181–187.

Silverman, M.M. (1989). Children of psychiatrically ill parents: A prevention perspective. *Hospital and Community Psychiatry, 40,* 1257–1265.

Smith, P.K., & Drew, L.M. (2002). Grandparenthood. In M.H. Bornstein (Ed.), *Handbook of parenting, Vol. 3: Being and becoming a parent* (2nd ed., pp. 141–172). Mahwah, NJ: Lawrence Erlbaum Associates.

Sneddon, J., Kerry, B.J., & Bant, W.P. (1981). The psychiatric mother and baby unit: 3-year study. *Practitioner, 225,* 1295–1300.

Solomon, J., & George, C. (1996). Defining the caregiving system: Toward a theory of caregiving. *Infant Mental Health Journal, 17,* 183–197.

Solomon, J., & George, C. (Eds.). (1999). *Attachment disorganization.* New York: Guilford Press.

Soskis, D.A., & Bowers, M.B. (1969). The schizophrenic experience. *The Journal of Nervous and Mental Disease, 149,* 443–449.

Sparrow, S., Balla, D., & Cicchetti, D. (2005). *Vineland Adaptive Behavior Scales* (Interview Edition, 2nd ed.). Circle Pines, MN: AGS Publishing.

Spielberger, C. (1973). *Manual for state-trait anxiety interview for children.* Palo Alto, CA: Consulting Psychologists Press.

Spinelli, M.G. (1999). Prevention of postpartum mood disorders. In L.J. Miller (Ed.), *Postpartum mood disorders* (pp. 212–235). Washington, DC: American Psychiatric Press.

Sroufe, L.A. (1995). *Emotional development: The organization of emotional life in the early years.* Cambridge, UK: Cambridge University Press.

Stanley, N., & Penhale, B. (1999). The mental health problems of mothers experiencing the child protection system. *Child Abuse Review, 8,* 34–45.

Steadman, H.J. & Monahan, J. (Eds.). (2001). *Violence and mental disorder: Developments in risk assessment.* Chicago: University of Chicago Press.

Steadman, H.J., Monahan, J., Appelbaum, P.S., Grisso, T., Mulvey, E.P., Roth, L.H., et al. (1994). Designing a new generation of risk assessment research. In J. Monahan & H.J. Steadman (Eds.), *Violence and mental disorder: Developments in risk assessment* (pp. 297–318). Chicago: University of Chicago Press.

Steiner, M., & Tam, W.Y.K. (1999). Postpartum depression in relation to other psychiatric disorders. In L.J. Miller (Ed.), *Postpartum mood disorders* (pp. 47–63). Washington, DC: American Psychiatric Press.

Stewart, D.E. (1984). Pregnancy and schizophrenia. *Canadian Family Physician, 30,* 1537–1541.

Straus, M.A. (2000). Conflict tactics scales. In K. Corcoran & J. Fischer (Eds.), *Measures for clinical practice: A sourcebook. Vol. 1: Couples, families, and children* (pp. 229–236). New York: Free Press.

Strauss, A.L., & Corbin, J. (1998). *Basics of qualitative research: Techniques and procedures for developing grounded theory.* Thousand Oaks, CA: Sage Publications.

Stubbe, D.E., Zahner, G.E., Goldstein, M.J., & Leckman, J.F. (1993). Diagnostic specificity of a brief measure of expressed emotion: A community study of children. *The Journal of Child Psychology and Psychiatry and Applied Disciplines, 34,* 139–154.

Sullivan, P.F., Neale, M.C., & Kendler, K.S. (2000). Genetic epidemiology of major depression: Review and meta-analysis. *American Journal of Psychiatry, 157,* 1552–1562.

Sullivan, P.M., & Knutson, J.F. (2000). Maltreatment and disabilities: A population-based epidemiologic study. *Child Abuse & Neglect: The International Journal, 24,* 1257–1273.

Symington, J., & Symington, N. (1999). *The clinical thinking of Wilfred Bion.* New York: Brunner-Routledge.

Tajima, E.A. (2000). The relative importance of wife abuse as a risk factor for violence against children. *Child Abuse and Neglect, 24,* 1383–1398.

Target, M., Shmueli-Goetz, Y., & Fonagy, P. (2003). Attachment representations in school-age children: The early development of the child attachment interview. *Journal of Child Psychotherapy, 29,* 171–186.

Tarullo, L.B., DeMulder, E.K., Ronsaville, D.S., Brown, E., & Radke-Yarrow, M. (1995). Maternal depression and maternal treatment of siblings as predictors of child psychopathology. *Developmental Psychology, 31,* 395–405.

Thorpe, K., Golding, J., MacGillivray, I., & Greenwood, R. (1991). Comparison of prevalence of depression in mothers of twins and mothers of singletons. *British Medical Journal, 302,* 875–878.

Tolan, P., Gorman-Smith, D., & Henry, D.B. (2003). The developmental ecology of urban males' youth violence. *Developmental Psychology, 39,* 274–281.

Totsika, V., & Sylva, K. (2004). The home observation for measurement of the environment revisited. *Child and Adolescent Mental Health, 9,* 25–35.

Trepper, T.S., & Barrett, M.J. (1989). *Systemic treatment of incest: A therapeutic handbook.* Bristol, PA: Taylor & Francis.

Triffleman, E., Marmar, C.R., Delucchi, K.L., & Ronfeldt, H. (1995). Childhood trauma and posttraumatic stress disorder in substance abuse inpatients. *Journal of Nervous and Mental Disease, 183,* 172–176.

Trocme, N. (1996). Development and preliminary evaluation of the Ontario Child Neglect Index. *Child Maltreatment, 1,* 145–155.

Uddenberg, N., & Engelsson, I. (1978). Prognosis of postpartum mental disturbance: A prospective study of primiparous women and their 4-1/2-year-old children. *Acta Psychiatrica Scandinavica, 58,* 201–212.

Venkataraman, M. (2005). *Parenting among mothers with bipolar disorder.* Unpublished doctoral dissertation, University of Illinois at Urbana-Champaign.

Viguera, A.C., Cohen, L.S., Baldessarini, R.J., & Nonacs, R. (2002). Managing bipolar disorder during pregnancy: Weighing the risks and benefits. *Canadian Journal of Psychiatry, 47,* 426–436.

Wahler, R.G. (1980). The insular mother: Her problems in parent–child treatment. *Journal of Applied Behavior Analysis, 13,* 207–219.

Walsh, F. (1999). *Spiritual resources in family therapy.* New York: Guilford Press.

Wannon, M. (1990). *Children's control attributions about controllable and uncontrollable events: Their relationship to stress-resiliency and psychological adjustment.* Unpublished doctoral dissertation, University of Rochester.

Wasserman, D.R., & Leventhal, J.M. (1993). Maltreatment of children born to cocaine-abusing mothers. *American Journal of Diseases of Children, 147,* 1324–1328.

Webster-Stratton, C., & Spitzer, A. (1991). Development, reliability, and validity of the daily telephone discipline interview: DDI. *Behavioral Assessment, 13,* 221–239.

Whiffen, V.E., & Gotlib, I.H. (1989). Infants of postpartum depressed mothers: Temperament and cognitive status. *Journal of Abnormal Psychology, 98,* 274–279.

Winnicott, D.W. (1949). *The ordinary devoted mother and her baby.* London: Tavistock Publications.

Winnicott, D.W. (1965*). The maturational process and the facilitating environment.* New York: International Universities Press.

Wisner, K.L., Peindl, K.S., Gigliotti, T., & Hanusa, B.H. (1999). Obsessions and compulsions in women with postpartum depression. *Journal of Clinical Psychiatry, 60,* 176–180.

Wolfe, D.A. (1991). *Preventing physical and emotional abuse of children.* New York: Guilford Press.

Wolfe, D.A. (1999). *Child abuse: Implications for child development and psychopathology.* Newbury Park, CA: Sage Publications.

Wyman, P.A., Cowen, E.L., Work, W.C., & Kerley, J.H. (1993). The role of children's future expectations in self-system functioning and adjustment to life stress: A prospective study of urban at-risk children. *Development and Psychopathology, 5,* 649–666.

Zeanah, C.H., & Benoit, D. (1995). Clinical applications of a parent perception interview in infant mental health. *Child and Adolescent Psychiatric Clinics of North America, 4,* 539–554.

Zeanah, C.H., Benoit, D., Barton, M., Regan, C., Hirshberg, L.M., & Lipsett, L.P. (1993). Representations of attachment in mothers and their one-year-old infants. *Journal of the American Academy of Child and Adolescent Psychiatry, 32,* 278–286.

Zeanah, C.H., & Boris, N. (2000). Disturbances and disorders of attachment in early childhood. In C.H. Zeanah (Ed.), *The handbook of infant mental health* (2nd ed., pp. 353–368). New York: Guilford Press.

Zeanah, C.H., Mammen, O.K., & Lieberman, A.F. (1993). Disorders of attachment. In C.H. Zeanah (Ed.), *Handbook of infant mental health* (pp. 332–349). New York: Guilford Press.

Zuravin, S.J. (1991). Unplanned childbearing and family size: Their relationship to child neglect and abuse. *Family Planning Perspectives, 23,* 155–161.

Instruments for Assessing Risk of Child Maltreatment

INSTRUMENTS FOR CHILDREN AND ADOLESCENTS

Construct	Instrument	Age range	Type, number of questions	Brief description	Citations
Attachment	The Attachment Doll-Play Interview (ADI) for Preschoolers	Preschool	Six story-stems describe separations and reunions of children and mothers.	Story-stems are enacted dramatically using a family of dolls including mother and child and, in some stories, fathers as well. Stories include depictions of separations and reunions at preschool, child falling and hurting self, and parents leaving for the movies and returning later.	Oppenheim, D. (1997). The Attachment Doll-Play Interview for Preschoolers. *International Journal of Behavioral Development, 20,* 681–697.
Behavior	The Child Behavior Checklist (CBCL)	2–18 years	The 112 items that comprise the CBCL are rated by parents or other close adults on a 3-point scale (0 = not true, 1 = somewhat or sometimes true, 2 = very true).	The CBCL yields a total score, two broad-band scores representing internalizing and externalizing dimensions of behavior and emotional problems, and scores for eight scales to assess withdrawn/depressed behavior, somatic complaints, social problems, anxious/depressed behavior, thought problems, at-	Achenbach T.M., & Rescorla. L.A. (2001). *Manual for the ASEBA School-Age Forms & Profiles.* Burlington, VT: University of Vermont, Research Center for Children, Youth, & Families. Dutra, L., Campbell, L., & Westen, D. (2004). Quantifying clinical judgment in the assessment of adolescent psychopathology: Re-

Measure	Age Range	Administration	Description	Reference
			tention problems, rule-breaking behavior, aggressive behavior.	liability, validity, and factor structure of the Child Behavior Checklist for clinician report. *Journal of Clinical Psychology, 60,* 65–85.
Child Behavior Questionnaire (CBQ)	3–7 years	Teachers or parents are asked to read a series of behaviors often displayed by children and respond on a 3-point scale.	The CBQ assesses dimensions of temperament including activity level, anger/frustration, attentional focusing, soothability, fear, and impulsivity.	Behar, L., & Stringfield, S. (1974). A behavior rating scale for the preschool child. *Developmental Psychology, 10,* 601–610.
Children's Depression Inventory (CDI)	6–17 years	27 items (self-report); 10–15 minutes	The CDI assesses cognitive, affective, and behavioral signs of depression in children and adolescents.	Fristad, M.A., Emery, B.L., & Beck, S.J. (1997). Use and abuse of the Children's Depression Inventory. *Journal of Consulting and Clinical Psychology, 65,* 699–702.
Beck Depression Inventory (BDI)	14 years and older	21 items (self-report); 5–10 minutes	The BDI measures characteristic attitudes and symptoms of depression.	Beck, A.T., Ward, C.H., Mendelson, M., Mock, J., & Erbaugh, J. (1961). An inventory for measuring depression. *Archives of General Psychiatry, 4,* 561–571.

(continued)

INSTRUMENTS FOR CHILDREN AND ADOLESCENTS *(continued)*

Construct	Instrument	Age range	Type, number of questions	Brief description	Citations
					Richter, P., Werner, J., Heerlien, A., Kraus, A., & Sauer, H. (1998). On the validity of the Beck Depression Inventory: A review. *Psychopathology, 31,* 160–168.
Development	Ages & Stages Questionnaires® (ASQ), Second Edition	4–60 months	Parent report; 19 items	The ASQ is a broad screening tool measuring development in five areas: communication, gross motor, fine motor, problem solving, and personal-social.	Bricker, D., & Squires, J. (1999). *Ages & Stages Questionnaires® (ASQ): A Parent-Completed, Child Monitoring System* (2nd ed.). Baltimore: Paul H. Brookes Publishing Co. Squires, J., Bricker, D., & Twombly, E. (2002). *Ages and Stages Questionnaires®: Social-Emotional (ASQ: SE): A parent-completed, child-monitoring system for social-emotional behaviors.* Baltimore: Paul H. Brookes Publishing Co.
	Bayley Scales of Infant Development, Third Edition (BTSD-III)	15 days–42 months	60 minutes	The BTSD-III includes a mental scale, motor scale, and behavior rating scale.	Bayley, N. (1993). *Bayley Scales of Infant Development* (2nd ed.). San Antonio, TX: The Psychological Corporation.

Category	Measure	Age range	Format	Description	Reference
	Vineland Adaptive Behavior Scales (VABS)	Birth–18 years, 11 months	Interview edition: 577 items (semi-structured); 60–90 minutes	The VABS measures adaptive behavior in the domains of communication, daily living skills, socialization, and motor skills.	Sparrow, S.S., Balla, D.A., & Cicchetti, D.V. (2005). *Vineland Adaptive Behavior Scales* (Interview ed., 2nd ed.). Circle Pines, MN: AGS Publishing.
Emotional and social impairment	Beck Youth Inventories of Emotional and Social Impairment	15–18 years, 1 month	30–60 minutes; self-report	The Beck Youth Inventories can be used separately or in combination to assess symptoms of depression, anxiety, anger, disruptive behavior, and self-concept.	Beck, J.S., Beck A.T., & Jolly, J. (2001). *Beck Youth Inventories of Emotional and Social Impairment manual.* San Antonio, TX: The Psychological Corporation.
Family stress	Adolescent Family Inventory of Life Events and Changes (A-FILE)	Adolescents	50 items; self-report	A-FILE measures adolescents' perceptions of the overall amount of stress experienced in their families and records life events and changes that adolescents perceive their families to have experienced during the past 12 months across 6 subscales.	McCubbin, H.I., Patterson, J., & Wilson, L. (1980). Family Inventory of Life Events and Changes (FILE). In H. McCubbin & A. Thompson (Eds.), *Family Assessment for Research and Practice.* Madison, WI: University of Wisconsin Press.
Intelligence	Stanford-Binet Intelligence Scale (SBIS), Fourth Edition	24 months–adult	15 subtests	The SBIS measures cognitive reasoning in the areas of verbal reasoning, quantitative reasoning, abstract/visual reasoning, and short-term memory	Laurent, J., Swerdlik, M., & Ryburn, M. (1992). Review of validity research on the Stanford-Binet Intelligence Scale (4th ed.). *Psychological Assessment, 4,* 102–112.

(continued)

INTRUMENTS FOR CHILDREN AND ADOLESCENTS *(continued)*

Construct	Instrument	Age range	Type, number of questions	Brief description	Citations
Trauma	Wechsler Preschool and Primary Scale of Intelligence-Revised (WPPSI-R)	4–6 years, 7 months	11 subtests administered by a professional (6 verbal and 5 performance)	The Verbal Scale measures language skills. The Performance Scale assesses nonverbal problem solving, perceptual organization, and visual-motor proficiency.	Sellers, A.H., Burns, W.J., & Guyrke, J. (2002). Differences in young children's IQs on the Wechsler Preschool and Primary Scale of Intelligence-Revised as a function of stratification variables. *Applied Neuropsychology, 9,* 65–73.
	Trauma Symptom Checklist for Children (TSCC); Version for younger children also available (TSCYC).	8–16 years	54 items on a 4-point scale; self-report	The TSCC is a measure of posttraumatic distress and related psychological symptomatology in children who have experienced traumatic events.	Briere, J. (1996). *Trauma Symptom Checklist for Children (TSCC) professional manual.* Odessa, FL: Psychological Assessment Resources. Briere, J., Johnson, K., Bissada, A., Damon, L., Crouch, J., Gil, E., Hanson, R., & Ernst, V. (2001). The Trauma Symptom Checklist for Young Children (TSCYC): Reliability and association with abuse exposure in a multi-site study. *Child Abuse & Neglect, 25,* 1001–1014.

INTRUMENTS FOR PARENTS, ADULTS, AND FAMILIES

Construct	Instrument	Age range	Type, number of questions	Brief description	Citations
Anxiety	State-Trait Anxiety Inventory (S-TAI)	Adults	40 multiple-choice questions, 10 minutes	The self-report measures state and trait anxiety.	Barnes, L.L., Harp, D., & Jung, W.S. (2002). Reliability generalization of scores on the Spielberger State-Trait Anxiety Inventory. *Educational and Psychological Measurement, 62*(4), 603–618.
Attachment	The Attachment Style Interview for Researchers & Clinicians		Structured interview	The Attachment Style Interview assesses characteristics of adults and young people in terms of the quality of close relationships, social support, and security of attachment style.	Bifulco, A., Figueiredo, B., Guedney, N., Gorman, L., Hayes, S., Muzik, M., et al. (2004). Maternal attachment style and depression associated with childbirth: Preliminary results from European/U.S. cross-cultural study. *British Journal of Psychiatry, 184*(Suppl. 46), s31–s37.

(continued)

INTRUMENTS FOR PARENTS, ADULTS, AND FAMILIES *(continued)*

Construct	Instrument	Age range	Type, number of questions	Brief description	Citations
	Adult Attachment Interview (AAI)		Semi-structured interview	The Adult Attachment Interview assesses characteristics of adults and young people in terms of the quality of close relationships, social support, and security of attachment style.	George, C., & Main, M. (1984). *Attachment interview for adults.* Unpublished manuscript, University of California at Berkeley. Hesse, E. (1999). The adult attachment interview: Historical and current perspectives. In J. Cassidy & P.R. Shaver (Eds.), *Handbook of attachment: Theory, research and clinical application* (pp. 395–433). New York: Guilford Press.
Attachment: Parent–Child Interaction Quality	CARE-INDEX	Birth to 24 months		The CARE-INDEX includes 5 minutes of videotaped adult–infant play interaction coded by facial expression, vocal expression, position and body contact, expression of affection, turn-taking, control, and choice of activity.	Crittenden, P.M. (1988). Relationships at risks. In J. Belsky & T. Nezworski (Eds.), *Clinical Implications of Attachment* (pp. 136–174). Hillsdale, NJ: Lawrence Erlbaum Associates.

Behavior: father to mother	Marital interactions	Observations of family interactions in lab setting	Families choose an area of disagreement and interact for 10 minutes. The families' total aversive behaviors are coded for information sharing, guiding interaction, control, agreement, criticism, and protest.	Webster-Stratton, C. (1990). Enhancing the effectiveness of self-administered videotape parent training for families with conduct-problem children. *Journal of Abnormal Child Psychology, 18*(5), 479–492.
Child abuse potential	CAP 3 Inventory	160-item, self-report	The CAP 3 is a screening tool for the detection of physical child abuse. The Clinical Scales assess distress, rigidity, unhappiness, problems with child and self, problems with family, and problems with others. The CAP Inventory contains lie, random response, and inconsistency scales.	Milner, J.S. et al. (1990). Childhood history of abuse and adult child abuse potential. *Journal of Family Violence, 5*(1), 15–34. Cerny, J.E., & Inouye, J. (2001). Utilizing the Child Abuse Potential Inventory in a community health nursing prevention program for child abuse. *Journal of Community Health Nursing, 18*(4), 199–211.
Child maltreatment	The Child Well-Being Scales	Rating scales completed by home observer	The Child Well-Being Scales include 43 separate dimensions including parenting role performance, familial capacities, child role performance, and child capacities.	Magura, S., & Moses, B. (1986). *Outcome measures for child welfare services: Theory and applications.* Washington, DC: Child Welfare League of America.

(continued)

INTRUMENTS FOR PARENTS, ADULTS, AND FAMILIES *(continued)*

Construct	Instrument	Age range	Type, number of questions	Brief description	Citations
Childhood experiences	Childhood Experience of Care and Abuse Interview		Semi-structured, retroactive interview	The Childhood Experience of Care and Abuse Interview assesses childhood experiences including neglect, antipathy, physical abuse, and sexual abuse.	Bifulco, A., Brown, G.W., & Harris, T. (1994). Childhood Experiences of Care and Abuse (CECA): A retrospective interview measure. *Child Psychology and Psychiatry, 35,* 1419–1435.
Conflict tactics	Conflict Tactics Scale		Couples	The Conflict Tactics Scale includes 80 items rated on a 7-point scale to assess the parent relationship with the child, parent partner's interactions with the child, and the interactions between the parent and the parent's partner.	Straus, M.A., & Gelles, R.J. (1990). *Physical violence in American families: Risk factors and adaptations to violence in 8,145 families.* New Brunswick, NJ: Transaction.
Depression	Beck Depression Inventory (BDI)	14 years and older	21 items (self-report), 5–10 minutes	The BDI measures characteristic attitudes and symptoms of depression	Beck, A.T., Ward, C.H., Mendelson, M., Mock, J., & Erbaugh, J. (1961). An inventory for measuring depression. *Archives of General Psychiatry, 4,* 561–571.

Richter, P., Werner, J., Heerlien, A., Kraus, A., & Sauer, H. (1998). On the validity of the Beck Depression Inventory: A review. *Psychopathology, 31*(3), 160–168.

Edinburgh Postnatal Depression Scale	Ten short statements answered by the mother	The Edinburgh Postnatal Depression Scale was developed to assist primary care health professionals to detect mothers suffering from postnatal depression.

Cox, J.L., Holden, J.M., & Sagovsky, R. (1987). Detection of postnatal depression: Development of the 10-item Edinburgh Postnatal Depression Scale. *British Journal of Psychiatry, 150,* 782–786.

Center for Epidemiological Studies Depression Scale (CESD)	20 items, self-report, items measured on 4-point scale indicating the degree of their occurrence in the past week	The CESD measures current level of depressive symptomatology, especially depressive affect.

Radloff, L.S., & Teri, L. (1999). Center for Epidemiological Studies Depression Scale [CES-D]. In A. Burns & S. Craig (Eds.), *Assessment scales in old age psychiatry.* London: Martin Dunitz.

(continued)

INTRUMENTS FOR PARENTS, ADULTS, AND FAMILIES *(continued)*

Construct	Instrument	Age range	Type, number of questions	Brief description	Citations
Emotional environment	Five Minute Speech Sample		Adult respondent and a relative respondent speak for 5 minutes in response to the prompt "I'd like you to speak for 5 minutes telling me what kind of person [relative's name] is and how the two of you get along."	The Five Minute Speech Sample distinguishes the nature of the respondent–relative environment by identifying emotions, feelings, and attitudes expressed by a respondent about a relative.	McCarty, C.A., & Weisz, J.R. (2002). Correlates of expressed emotion in mothers of clinically-referred youth: An examination of the Five-Minute Speech Sample. *Journal of Child Psychology and Psychiatry and Allied Disciplines, 43*(6), 759–768.
Family relationships	Family Adaptability and Cohesion Scales IV (FACES IV)		Family member; 20 negatively and positively stated questions scored on a Likert-type scale	FACES IV assesses an individual's perceived levels of family cohesion, adaptability, and level of functioning.	Franklin, C., Streeter, C.L., & Springer, D.W. (2001). Validity of the FACES IV Family Assessment Measure. *Research on Social Work Practice, 11*(5), 576–596.
	Perceived Family Burden Scale (PFBS)		Family member of an adult with schizophrenia	The PFBS measures behaviors of patients with schizophrenia to distinguish between the objective and	Levene, J.E., Lancee, W.J., & Seeman, M.V. (1996). The Perceived Family Burden Scale: Measurement and

	Eco-maps	Completed with a mental health worker	subjective components of family burden. Eco-maps is a visual tool of a family's interactions.	validation. *Schizophrenia and Research, 22*(2), 151–157. Hartman, A. (1978). Diagrammatic assessment of family relationships. *Social Casework, 59,* 465–476.
	Genogram		Family diagrams that generally follow the conventions of genealogical charts are used to identify meaningful familial patterns.	Hartman, A. (1978). Diagrammatic assessment of family relationships. *Social Casework, 59,* 465–476. McGoldrick, M., Gerson, R., & Shellenberger, S. (1999). *Genograms: Assessment and intervention.* New York: W.W. Norton.
Home safety	Home Safety Checklist	Child protection workers	The Home Safety Checklist identifies 42 elements of home safety to discuss with parents such as not storing poisonous household products in jars, having emergency numbers near the phone, and placing beds away from windows.	Illinois Department of Children and Family Services, Office of the Inspector General. (1999). *Home safety checklist.* Chicago: Author.

(continued)

INTRUMENTS FOR PARENTS, ADULTS, AND FAMILIES (*continued*)

Construct	Instrument	Age range	Type, number of questions	Brief description	Citations
Infant–caregiver interaction	Infant-Caregiver Interaction Scale (ICIS)		Observation of parent–child interactions	The ICIS looks at infant and caregiver behaviors during feeding and play interactions and in the environment.	Munson, L.J., & Odom, S.L. (1997). Rating scales that measure parent–infant interaction. *Newsletter of the Australian Early Intervention Association (NSW Chapter) Inc. 5*(1), 13–24. Odom, S.L., Schertz, H., Munson, L.J., & Brown, W. (2004). Assessing social competence. In M. McLean, D. Bailey, & M. Wolery (Eds.), *Assessing infants and preschoolers with special needs* (3rd ed). Columbus, OH: Merrill.
Intelligence	Wechsler Adult Intelligence Scales (WAIS)	Ages 16 and older		The WAIS includes verbal IQ, performance IQ, and full scale IQ tests.	Taub, G.E. (2001). A confirmatory analysis of the Wechsler Adult Intelligence Scale-Third Edition: Is the verbal/performance discrepancy justified? *Practical Assessment, Research and Evaluation, 7*(22), 1–9.

Life stress	Life Stress Scale	39 items, self-report on a 4-point scale	The Life Stress Scale assesses the level of disruption that various situations have on the lives of adults.	Egeland, B., Breitenbucher, M., & Rosenberg, D. (1980). Prospective study of the significance of life stress in the etiology of child abuse. *Journal of Consulting and Clinical Psychology, 48*, 195–205.
Parenting	Screening for Problem Parenting	20-item scale	Screening for Problem Parenting assesses social support and parenting attitudes.	Avison, W.R., Turner, R.J., & Noh, S. (1986). Screening for problem parenting: Preliminary evidence of a promising instrument. *Child Abuse and Neglect, 10*(2), 157–170.
	Adult-Adolescent Parenting Inventory	Self-report	The Adult-Adolescent Parenting Inventory is a 32-item instrument that assesses parenting strengths and weaknesses including developmental expectations of children, empathy, belief in the use of corporal punishment, and reversing child–parent roles.	Bavolek, S.J. (1984). *Handbook for the Adult-Adolescent Parenting Inventory.* Eau Claire, WI: Family Development Associates.

(continued)

INTRUMENTS FOR PARENTS, ADULTS, AND FAMILIES *(continued)*

Construct	Instrument	Age range	Type, number of questions	Brief description	Citations
Parenting skills and home environment	Infant/Toddler Home Observation for the Measurement of the Environment (HOME) Inventory; Early Childhood HOME Inventory; Middle Childhood HOME Inventory; Early Adolescent HOME Inventory	Infant–toddler; early childhood; middle childhood; early adolescence		HOME assesses parental responsivity, acceptance of child, organization of the environment, learning materials, parental involvement, and variety in experience; and the quality and quantity of stimulation and support available to a child in the home environment. The focus is on the child in the environment and child as recipient of inputs for objects, events, and transactions occurring in connection with the family surroundings.	Bradley, R.H., Corwyn, R.F., Caldwell, B.M., Whiteside-Mansell, L., Wasserman, G.A., Walker, T.B., & Mink, I.T. (2000). Measuring the home environments of children in early adolescence. *Journal of Research on Adolescence, 10,* 247–289.

Psychopathology in mother–child interactions	The Bethlem Mother–Infant Interaction Scale (BMIS)	Mother–infant observation by professional of post-partum women with severe psychiatric illness	The Scale assesses the appropriateness of the mother's caregiving behaviors, including her ability to elicit and maintain visual, physical, and vocal contact with the baby, the sensitivity and responsiveness of her mood, her ability to maintain routine care of the baby, and the assessment by staff of any risk to the baby through impulse or "neglect."	Hipwell, AE., & Kumar, R. (1996). Maternal psychopathology and prediction of outcome based on mother–infant interaction ratings. *British Journal of Psychiatry, 169*(5), 655–661.
Social support	Inventory of Socially Supportive Behaviors (ISSB)	Self-report questionnaire; 10 minutes	The ISSB assesses a person's social support network in various areas	Barrera, M.J., & Ainlay, S.I. (1983). The structure of social support: A conceptual and empirical analysis. *Journal of Community Psychology, 11*, 133–143. Barrera, M.J., Sandler, I.N., & Ramsay, T.B. (1981). Preliminary development of a scale of social support: Studies on college students. *Journal of Community Psychology, 9*, 435–447.

(continued)

INTRUMENTS FOR PARENTS, ADULTS, AND FAMILIES *(continued)*

Construct	Instrument	Age range	Type, number of questions	Brief description	Citations
	Childhood Social Network Questionnaire (CSNQ)		Personal history, sibling support		Feiring, C., Taska, L., & Lewis, M. (1998). Social support and children's and adolescents' adaptation to sexual abuse. *Journal of Interpersonal Violence, 13*(2), 240–260.
	Maternal Social Support Index (MSSI)		Self-report; 21-item questionnaire	Qualitative and quantitative aspects of a mother's social support are examined.	Pascoe, J.M., Lalongo, N.S., Horn, W.F., Reinhart, M.A., & Perradatto, D. (1988). The reliability and validity of the maternal social support index. *Family Medicine, 20*(4), 271–276.

Appendix B

Resources for Clinicians

MENTAL ILLNESS AND PARENTING

Apfel, R.J., & Handel, M.H. (1993). *Madness and loss of motherhood: Sexuality, reproduction, and long-term mental illness.* Washington, DC: American Psychiatric Press.

Cleaver, H., Unell, I., & Aldgate, J. (1999). *Children's needs—Parenting capacity. The impact of parental mental illness, problem alcohol and drug use, and domestic violence on children's development.* London: The Stationary Office.

Göpfert, M., Webster, J., and Seeman, M.V. (Eds.). (2004). *Parental psychiatric disorder: Distressed parents and their families* (2nd ed.). Cambridge, England: Cambridge University Press.

Hendrick, V. (Ed.). (2006). *Treatment of psychiatric disorders in pregnancy and the postpartum: Principles and treatment.* Totowa, NJ: Humana Press.

Holley, T.E., & Holley, J. (1997). *My mother's keeper: A daughter's memoir of growing up in the shadow of schizophrenia.* New York: William Morrow.

Lyden, J. (1997). *Daughter of the Queen of Sheba.* Boston: Houghton Mifflin.

Marsh, D.T. (1998). *Serious mental illness and the family: The practitioner's guide.* Somerset, NJ: John Wiley & Sons.

Murray, L., & Cooper, P.J. (Eds). *Postpartum depression and child development.* New York: Guilford Press.

Nicholson, J., Biebel, K., Hinden, B., Henry, A., & Stier, L. (2001). *Critical issues for parents with mental illness and their families* (KEN01 – 0109). Rockville, MD: Center for Mental Health Services, Substance Abuse and Mental Health Services Administration.

Nicholson, J., Henry, A.D., Clayfield, J., & Phillips, S. (2001). *Parenting well when you're depressed: A complete resource for maintaining a healthy family.* Oakland, CA: New Harbinger Publications.

Patterson, J.P. (1996). *Sweet mystery: A Southern memoir of family alcoholism, mental illness, and recovery.* New York: Farrar, Straus & Giroux.

CHILD DEVELOPMENT AND ATTACHMENT

Bowlby, J. (1988). *A secure base: Clinical applications of attachment theory.* London: Routledge.

Cassidy, J., & Shaver, P.R. (Eds.). (1999). *Handbook of attachment: Theory, research, and clinical applications.* New York: Guilford Press.

Damon, W., & Eisenberg, N. (Eds.). (2006). *Handbook of child psychology: Vol. 3. Social, emotional, and personality development* (6th ed.). Hoboken, NJ: John Wiley & Sons.

Damon, W., Sigel, I., & Renninger, K.A. (Eds.). (2006). *Handbook of child psychology: Vol. 4. Child psychology in practice* (6th ed.). Hoboken, NJ: John Wiley & Sons.

Lieberman, A.F. (1993). *The emotional life of the toddler.* New York: Free Press.

Solomon, J., & George, C. (Eds.). (1999). *Attachment disorganization.* New York: Guilford Press.

Sroufe, L.A. (1995). *Emotional development: The organization of emotional life in the early years.* Cambridge, England: Cambridge University Press.

CHILD MALTREATMENT, TRAUMA, AND VIOLENCE

Dubowitz, H. (1999). *Neglected children: Research, practice, and policy.* Thousand Oaks, CA: Sage Publications.

Feerick, M., Knutson, J., Trickett, P., & Flanzer, S. (2006). *Child abuse and neglect: Definitions, classifications, and a framework for research.* Baltimore: Paul H. Brookes Publishing Co.

Feerick, M., & Silverman, G. (2006). *Children exposed to violence.* Baltimore: Paul H. Brookes Publishing Co.

Helfer, M.E., Kempe, R.S., & Krugman, R.D. (1997). *The battered child* (5th ed.). Chicago: University of Chicago Press.

Lieberman, A.F., & Van Horn, P. (2005). *Don't hit my mommy! A manual for child–parent psychotherapy with young witnesses of family violence.* Washington, DC: Zero to Three.

Osofsky, J.D., & Fenichel, E. (1996). *Islands of safety: Assessing and treating young victims of violence.* Washington, DC: ZERO TO THREE: National Center for Infants, Toddlers and Families.

Steadman, H.J., & Monahan, J. (2001). *Violence and mental disorder: Developments in risk assessment.* Chicago: University of Chicago Press.

ASSESSMENT

Dulcan, M.K., Martini, D.R., & Lake, M. (2003). *Concise guide to child and adolescent psychiatry* (3rd ed.). Washington, DC: American Psychiatric Publishing.

Gambrill, E. (2005). *Critical thinking in clinical practice: Improving the quality of judgments and decisions* (2nd ed.). Hoboken, NJ: John Wiley & Sons.

Goldstein, J., Freud, A., & Solnit, A.J. (1973). *Beyond the best interests of the child.* London: Collier Macmillan.

Goldstein, J, Solnit, A.J., Goldstein, S., & Freud, A. (1998). *The best interests of the child: The least detrimental alternative.* New York: Free Press.

Grisso, T. (2002). *Evaluating competencies: Forensic assessments and instruments.* (2nd ed.) New York: Springer.

Herman, S.P. (1997). Practice parameters for the American Academy of Child and Adolescent Psychiatry: Child custody evaluation. *Journal of the American Academy of Child and Adolescent Psychiatry, 36*(Suppl.10), 57S–68S.

Jordan, C., & Franklin, C. (Eds.). (2003). *Clinical assessment for social workers: Quantitative and qualitative methods* (2nd ed.). Chicago: Lyceum Books.

Reder, P., & Lucey, C. (Eds.). (1995). *Assessment of parenting: Psychiatric and psychological contributions.* London: Routledge.

Sattler, J.M. (2002). *Assessment of children: Behavioral and clinical applications* (4th ed.). La Mesa, CA: Jerome M. Sattler.

Simon, R.I., & Gold, L.H. (Eds.). (2004). *Textbook of forensic psychiatry: The clinician's guide.* Washington, DC: American Psychiatric Publishing.

Index

Page numbers followed by *f* indicate figures; those followed by *t* indicate tables.

183